MAKING
MEANING IN
OLDER AGE

MAKING MEANING IN OLDER AGE

Bringing Together the Pieces of Your Life

Annette M. Lane, RN, PhD & Marlette B. Reed, BEd, MA

MAKING MEANING IN OLDER AGE
Copyright © 2017 by Dr. Annette Lane and Marlette Reed

Scripture quotations marked (TLB) are taken from The Living Bible copyright © 1971. Used by permission of Tyndale House Publishers, Inc., Carol Stream, Illinois 60188. All rights reserved. Scripture quotations marked (GNT) are from the Good News Translation in Today's English Version—Second Edition Copyright © 1992 by American Bible Society. Used by Permission. Scripture quotations marked (RSV) are from the Revised Standard Version of the Bible, copyright © 1946, 1952, and 1971 the Division of Christian Education of the National Council of the Churches of Christ in the United States of America. Used by permission. All rights reserved. Scripture quotations from THE MESSAGE. Copyright © by Eugene H. Peterson 1993, 1994, 1995, 1996, 2000, 2001, 2002. Used by permission of NavPress. All rights reserved. Represented by Tyndale House Publishers, Inc. Scripture quotations taken from the New American Standard Bible® (NASB), Copyright © 1960, 1962, 1963, 1968, 1971, 1972, 1973, 1975, 1977, 1995 by The Lockman Foundation. Used by permission. www.Lockman.org. Scripture quotations marked (NIV) are taken from the Holy Bible, New International Version®, NIV®. Copyright © 1973, 1978, 1984. 2011 by Biblica, Inc.™ Used by permission of Zondervan. All rights reserved worldwide. www.zondervan.com The "NIV" and "New International Version" are trademarks registered in the United States Patent and Trademark Office by Biblica, Inc.™ Scripture quotations marked (KJV) taken from the Holy Bible, King James Version, which is in the public domain. Scripture quotations are taken from the Holy Bible, New Living Translation, copyright ©1996, 2004, 2007, 2013, 2015 by Tyndale House Foundation. Used by permission of Tyndale House Publishers, Inc., Carol Stream, Illinois 60188. All rights reserved. Scripture taken from the New Century Version®. Copyright © 2005 by Thomas Nelson. Used by permission. All rights reserved. Scripture quotations marked "Phillips" are taken from The New Testament in Modern English, copyright © 1958, 1959, 1960 J.B. Phillips and 1947, 1952, 1955, 1957 The Macmillian Company, New York. Used by permission. All rights reserved.

ISBN: 978-1-4866-1432-5 Printed in Canada

Word Alive Press
131 Cordite Road, Winnipeg, MB R3W 1S1
www.wordalivepress.ca

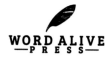
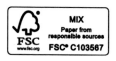

MIX
Paper from
responsible sources
FSC www.fsc.org **FSC® C103567**

Library and Archives Canada Cataloguing in Publication

Lane, Annette M., 1962-, author
    Making meaning in older age : bringing together the pieces of your life / Annette M. Lane, RN, PhD & Marlette B. Reed, BEd, MA.

Issued in print and electronic formats.
ISBN 978-1-4866-1432-5 (softcover).--ISBN 978-1-4866-1433-2 (ebook)

    1. Aging--Religious aspects--Christianity. 2. Older Christians--Religious life. 3. Older people--Family relationships. I. Reed, Marlette B., 1962-, author II. Title.

BV4580.L36 2017   248.8'5   C2016-907914-7
                                                          C2016-907915-5

DEDICATION

To the older adults we have worked with over the years, our sincere gratitude for your examples of courage, resilience, and humor.

and

To my wonderful husband Dave: the years of your support, companionship, and laughter has carried me. (Annette)

To Brian and Jon and Erin: Love you so much. (Marlette)

CONTENTS

Foreword

...God has planted eternity in the hearts of men...
—Ecclesiastes 3:11 (TLB)

A satisfactory life has to be crafted*... one must see (old) age for what it is—a different mode and decide what one wants from it,* in it.... *An artist friend says if a man painted one masterpiece in his entire life, it was worth all his other effort.*
—Michael Drury, 1988, italics ours

Ever more people today have the means to live, but no meaning to live for.
—Viktor E. Frankl
Holocaust survivor and Austrian psychiatrist
(Brainy Quotes, 2016a)

We confess, we are meaning junkies! That is, for as long as we can remember, we have been interested in, and indeed driven by, the need for meaning in our lives. As a young girl, lying on our home's front lawn, Marlette remembers looking up at the clouds and wondering, "What does this all mean?"

The passion for meaning influenced our careers and resulted in our work with individuals, often at the lowest points in their lives (e.g. dying and death, refugee camp nursing, working with individuals with dementia and their caregivers, crisis counseling). And, in our personal and work experiences, we have come to recognize the poignancy of Viktor Frankl's quote. Although individuals in developed countries have far more amenities and comforts than a century ago, meaning in life seems far more elusive, sometimes even absent.

Ironically, some people find that meaning is absent in places where it should be present (such as in faith communities), and others find vigorous meaning in unexpected places or situations, such as in a hospice, where a loved one is dying ("I'll never be the same again," stated one woman, referring to the surprising growth she experienced accompanying her dying mother through that transition).

This is not a theological book, per se. But it is a spiritual one—one which deals with matters of the soul, often so prominent for older adults, and those who love them. There will be biblical references throughout. However, we have purposefully left in-depth discussion of the scriptural foundations of this book's concepts for Chapter Six; we would like to utilize current languaging and research to describe the journey, and then bring in the age-old truths of the Bible, which underpin psychology, later on. With current information and discussion on this subject in the first part of the book, we believe you will have more finely focused spiritual lenses to broaden your vision and deepen your appreciation of the scriptures discussed in the lengthy end chapter.

Throughout the six chapters, a number of themes will be expressed; they will recur, as they are, we believe, so critical to fulfillment during this stage of life. Here they are:

- A deep sense of meaning is integral to most human beings.
- While meaning is vital to most people, it is for older adults even more significant.
- Meaning is both theoretical (a paradigm through which one processes life, such as spirituality or religion) and practical (the outworking of that inner paradigm through commitments and activities).
- Meaning can be *made*, in that one can actively develop meaning intellectually, spiritually, and socially—through activities chosen, associations developed, and even thinking processes adopted.
- There is meaning in *being* (the inherent value of creation and humanity) and in *doing* (how we choose to live our lives).
- Having meaning enhances physical and mental health and life satisfaction.
- The life experience of older adults, rarely written down, is tacit knowledge—that which is real, important, but difficult to communicate through the written word. The tacit knowledge of older adults is essential in the perseverance of our civilization. And we

think it is imperative, so that our society remains civilized!

- The mistakes of our lives can be redeemed, and a masterpiece can emerge from that which was originally damaged. Two metaphors will be used in this book: the tapestry that looks messy from one side, but is wonderfully layered and complex on the other, and the Japanese art of kintsugi, where broken pottery is repaired by fusing fractured pieces using precious metals of gold, silver, or platinum. The brokenness is incorporated into the restored piece and that piece is made even more beautiful than it was before the wounding. There is a redemptive theme that runs through the Scriptures, and God is in the business (with our cooperation) of weaving that theme through our lives, to produce tapestries, or vases, of beauty.

Please also be alert to other concepts, such as resilience, self-transcendence, and wresting and resting, nourishment of the soul, lenses of the soul (spiritual lenses), as well as chronic sorrow.

We introduce various case studies in order to illustrate our points. Some of the examples are composites of individuals with whom we have worked. Any resemblance to individuals you might know is coincidental, as identifying details have been removed. As well, there will be questions to ponder and activities, if you wish to take action on what you read, at the end of each chapter.

We openly confess that while we seek life's essence fervently, we have not figured out this whole area of meaning. And yet, we believe, as Michael Drury says, that older age needs to be crafted, and that if one paints, constructs, or produces one masterpiece in his or her lifetime, this individual has done well! That priceless work of art comes in all kinds of forms, including the well-formed character of one who has walked with God through the years and has had their life shaped into something that bears resemblance to their Companion.

As we offer what we hope are helpful ideas towards finding meaning, we recognize that we are continuously in this process; we never fully arrive, but meaning comes through the process, not just in the destination. This book is a guidebook—a map, if you will—for those approaching their latter years, and for those in them. It is also for adult children of elderly parents. We hope that it will be both informative as well as a gentle, spiritual prod to deepen your capacity to find, and sustain, meaning. Thank you for journeying with us into this daunting but fruitful territory!

chapter one

WHAT DOES IT MEAN TO HAVE MEANING?

These are the words of the Philosopher, David's son, who was king in Jerusalem. It is useless, useless, said the Philosopher. Life is useless, all useless.
—Ecclesiastes 1:1–2 (GNT)

So many people walk around with a meaningless life. They seem half-asleep, even when they they're busy doing things they think are important.
—Morrie Schwartz
Professor and Author
(Goodreads, 2016a)

What is meaning and why is it so important? Why, in our wealthy North American society, is meaning so difficult to find and hold onto? As noted by author Morrie Schwartz, people are furiously busy yet seem disconnected. How is it that individuals are so busy yet experience such pointlessness? If an individual finds meaning missing in her life, how can she find it?

Within this chapter, we attempt to unravel what meaning is by examining its qualities. We also consider how meaning is tied to self-identity, both in terms of who we are as people and how we express meaning. We address why meaning is so important and the impact that lacking meaning has upon a person. This beginning chapter then sets the stage for understanding meaning and meaning-making in later life, covered in the remainder of this book. Throughout the chapters, we will offer some theoretical information, but hopefully many more practical ideas. Our hope is that you will look at meaning-making in a different light and, within that, find ways to make and sustain meaning in your life, as well as the lives of beloved aging individuals.

WHAT DOES THE TERM MEANING MEAN?

The term *meaning* is actually quite difficult to define. Perhaps a useful place to begin to grasp its depth is to suggest what it is not. Although a related term, meaning is not just purpose. Meaning is imbued with an emotional quality that is sometimes lacking in a purpose. Countless loads of laundry have been done without the enrichment of the soul: purposeful activity, but lacking spiritual and emotional meaning.

Further, meaning is not interchangeable with happiness, although happiness may be a byproduct of having meaning. Also, having meaning is not necessarily easy. It is often assumed that an individual who has meaning in his life is simply lucky; he has a gift—of artistic, athletic, or intellectual ability—and hence an advantage over the rest of us who have to find our way in this world, looking for meaning. Life and its meaning have been handed to him on a silver platter. As will become clearer throughout this book, meaning-making is often laborious.

And while meaning in life can be tied to identity, self-identity and meaning are not synonymous. So the term *meaning* is connected with purpose, and meaning resonates deep within the souls of individuals; it can be called life's essence. Whatever is found to be meaningful is profoundly significant and of value to the individual. That being said, the term meaning is still somewhat slippery. How do we appropriately describe the depth and breadth of this important concept? C.S. Lewis said, "Reason is the natural order of truth; but imagination is the organ of meaning" (Brainy Quotes, 2016b). As we try to work with the concept of meaning using reason, order, and truth, please use your imagination to grab hold of what life's essence is to you, to your soul.

Ethereal and Existential Components

To start examining meaning, it may be helpful to divide meaning into three components: the ethereal and existential; meaning in connection; and the practical working out of meaning in day-to-day living. The ethereal aspect involves the spiritual nature of meaning. It includes the intangible and less obvious facets of a person, such as life paradigm or philosophy, religious faith or spirituality (Haugan, 2014a; Morgan & Farsides, 2009). As difficult as the word *meaning* is to define, so is the word *spiritual*. Power Thesaurus (2016) lists 470 synonyms for this word! Succinctly, the spiritual dimension of meaning is about values and guides to help one act in accordance with one's values, a way of looking at and processing the world and one's experiences within it (the lenses of the soul), nourishment of the soul, and wresting and resting.

VALUES AND GUIDES

From early life, parents teach their children what is important, and how to live within that system of values. For instance, early in a child's development, he learns the word "no!" Initially, it comes from his parents to protect him from placing his tiny, vulnerable hand on the stove. Then, he learns the word in the context of others: "no!" means not hitting others. While his safety is valuable, so is the safety of others. (Suffice it to say, this developing soul learns the word "no!" in the context of his own expression of what he wants or doesn't want.) Kindness towards others, honesty, empathy—all these values and more are taught within the home. Over time, this child internalizes the values taught; sometimes he rejects them in favor of others. However, in healthy development, the older child chooses to behave morally from a spiritual center within him; he does what is right and values what is good from within him, not simply because if he does what is not good, he will be punished. His values will guide him throughout his life, shape his choices, and help him to know who he is in relation to others around him. He will have developed *character* that will prepare him to face life as an adult.[1]

Besides the family of origin, the guides to living out these values come from a number of sources. They can

---

1 As a side note, there are many people who are adults chronologically but do not possess the character of mature adulthood. They still respond as children when they do not get what they want and will choose to do wrong if it is advantageous to them.

come from spiritual texts: did you know that most of the religions of the world have a variation of the Golden Rule within their written spiritual guides? "Do unto others as you would have them do unto you" is expressed in Buddhism this way: "Hurt not others in ways that you yourself would find hurtful" (Udana-Varga *5:18*). And in Taoism, the Golden Rule is expressed as follows: "Regard your neighbor's gain as your own gain, and your neighbor's loss as your own loss" (Tai Shang Kan Ying P'ien, 213–218) (Plumadore & Muehlherr, 2009). Words to live by!

The guides to spiritual values can also be, as alluded to before, parental and family beliefs, maxims, and mottos. In our family of origin, our father spoke regularly this maxim: "If you don't have something good to say about someone, don't say anything." Lovely, and in some ways very true! Except that it did not allow for truth-telling and honest communication when that was needed. Maxims can be guides, but because of their concise nature they are not always applicable in every circumstance.

Mentors are also spiritual guides, and their value cannot be overstated. By definition, a mentor is an experienced person who advises a less experienced one (Merriam Webster, 2016). These can be more formal arrangements, such as a new employee being mentored by a more seasoned one in a work setting. An effective mentor not only shows the mentee the ropes, so to speak, but also guides the new employee in the values of the organization, in what he needs to know so that his experience in the company is a good one. In Chapter Five, we will talk more about the importance of older adults *having* mentors, as well as *being* mentors to others.

Also, an organized community of faith can provide guidance and values for people. The values for living are communicated regularly: taught by the leaders; spoken out by the people through prayers, creeds, and liturgy; and internalized through public worship. Its value for meaning is also tied to community—connection—which will be spoken about briefly. These values and guides can provide structure in daily living, and in particular, be extremely comforting in times of major change or crisis.

LENSES THROUGH WHICH TO PROCESS THE WORLD

An important part of the spiritual dimension of living is that a life paradigm gives one a lens through which to process the world, and life events (Haugan, 2014b). The values and guides help individuals to act in ways that are beneficial for self and others. This spiritual lens gives one the framework through which to interpret and manage what life brings. How does one cope with disaster? After 9/11 in New York (2001), American churches were full to overflowing. The people were grabbing hold of "glasses" (which perhaps had been set on many night tables in the nation) through which to process such a devastating event. Though church attendance dropped off in the months following, the aftereffects of 9/11—fear, PTSD—have not.

Prior to 9/11, sociologist Barry Glassner spoke of fear in the U.S. in his book *The Culture of Fear: Why Americans Are Afraid of the Wrong Things* (1999). He cited that three out of four Americans were more fearful than they had been twenty years earlier, but argued that the actual risk of danger was not greater; rather, it was the public's perception of danger that had been heightened.

Glassner updated his book in 2009 to acknowledge the impact of 9/11. Certainly, one could argue that the events of 9/11 exacerbated fear. Both books, however, illustrate that difficult life experiences test our paradigms: our spiritual lenses may become cloudy. We may question our own paradigms by asking existential questions. Why am I (still) here? What is the purpose of my life? Is there life after death? Our understanding about life may not be sufficient to incorporate the experience; we may struggle to find meaning, we may fear, or even despair. The challenge for individuals in crisis then becomes how to put on the glasses of one's youth or change the prescription of the lenses (at least somewhat) so that one can find peace. It may mean grabbing hold of a maxim that can sustain: "Everything happens for a reason," said one man after a loss in his life. Though he did not know the reason (and Marlette, as his workplace chaplain, did not find this axiom personally helpful), it gave him peace.

Sadly, for some the stress upon the paradigm is too great and the lenses are shattered. This condition can occur when the life events are so dramatic that the soul is traumatized; if there is no help in that state of brokenness, severe mental illness can ensue and suicide, tragically, can result. There is growing recognition in North America that veterans of military service may suffer from Post-Traumatic Stress Disorder and need help to either have their lenses fixed or receive a new set of lenses, through opportunity to work through the horrors experienced, a safe place to grieve, balm and nourishment for the soul through spiritual and physical practices, and, sometimes, a significantly altered paradigm. In all of this, a sense of *meaning* has to be reestablished.

Annette M. Lane and Marlette B. Reed

NOURISHMENT FOR THE SOUL

A number of people have referred to North American society as soulless, including former Pope John Paul II. The press for more and more material goods, lengthy workweeks, hours spent in front of the television, and being packed into high-density cities like bees in a hive, yet not knowing one's own neighbors, create lives filled with stress, tedium, and isolation from others and from self. The soul, the essence of a person, can feel empty, restless, and troubled.

One of the key tasks for a young child is to learn to self-soothe. Early on in her development, when she feels anxiety and cannot be held by a parent (perhaps her parents are away for the evening), she calms herself through holding on to a teddy bear. She is not in physical danger, but the fears of her soul are put to rest through holding on to something that gives her comfort.

This is the beginning of developing mechanisms—whether psychological (such as sayings to recite when one feels they are running on empty), physical (going for a good run can be good for the body and soul) or spiritual (sitting quietly in an empty place of worship, or soaking in the sun while sitting along the bank of a burbling brook)—to calm the restlessness, reconnect a person with meaning, and nourish the soul throughout life.

Later in life, the ability to self-soothe (though this term is generally applied to young children) is vital. As different supports are lost through death, illness, and financial constraints, the value of being able to nourish one's own soul cannot be underestimated.

WRESTING AND RESTING

The word *wrest* can have a negative connotation and is sometimes used to connote usurping, or extorting. We are not using the term here in that way. Rather, we'd like to use *wrest* with the idea of seizing, grabbing hold of, or squeezing. In the context of meaning, this involves grabbing hold of lenses through which to process life, squeezing out meaning when life puts the squeeze on you, and seizing the day. "Carpe diem," a phrase used by Roman poet Horace, was famously quoted by actor Robin Williams in the 1989 movie *The Dead Poet's Society*: "Carpe diem. Seize the day, boys. Make your lives extraordinary." It is in this sense that we utilize the word *wrest*: making life extraordinary, making your life a work of art.

In some ways, resting is the opposite of this. It is the letting go—of past hurts, of disappointments, of future plans when it seems they are not to be. How does one know when it is time to wrest, or when it is time to rest? There are no easy answers. And we suspect it can be different for each person. For instance, a cancer diagnosis can be, for some, the motivation to wrest—to grab hold of—every opportunity for treatment. This may mean, for this person, an improvement in health, entering a clinical trial that may help in the research for new treatment options in the future, and/or the opportunity to test her mettle in ways she never anticipated. For another, it may mean *resting*—a letting go of anticipated plans, trusting in the ways of God, and an opportunity to model grace.

The two concepts are not mutually exclusive. Using the example of a cancer diagnosis, one may wrest and rest at the same time: being part of a new medication trial and accessing all the treatments recommended by the oncology team, but trusting in God for that which is out of one's control. One man, just hearing of his devastating cancer diagnosis, said, "No matter what happens, I have Christ. So if I live, I win; if I die, I win." As he availed himself of all the treatment options, he wrested; as he acknowledged that he could we die, he trusted in God and rested. This dual action approach can be a complex internal dance of wresting to seize meaning, control, and mastery; but when fear threatens to consume, the individual shifts internally to *rest* in the face of that which he cannot control. More on these concepts throughout the pages of this book.

CONNECTION

Meaning also involves connection to others. It can be inherent in belonging to one's family ("You're a Johnson; be proud!") or in culture. This inherited meaning can be both a blessing—a sense of identity without having to work for it—and a constraint. After attending an Asian wedding, Marlette exclaimed to an attendee, "I was born into the wrong culture! I'd like to join yours!" She was so moved with the sense of community, the identity, and the belonging of the individuals in that group. The attendee said to her, "Yes, there are some good things, but it's not all good, you know. There are expectations, assumptions, nosiness..."

Connection to one's ancestors can place one in a larger picture. This can be truly revelatory to the one searching for one's forbearers in the land of their origin. Some may appreciate the connection (and what it entails) more than others.

Our parents emigrated from the Netherlands to Canada prior to the birth of their children. While we as children were always proud that our parents were immigrants (we thought it took plenty of jam to come from another country!), the actual country from which they came was not important. The stories they told us of their lives in Holland were nice, but not particularly significant (with the exception of their WW2 experiences). However, when both of our parents passed away in a span of four years, we wanted to go to the Netherlands to understand from whence we came. We not only went to the Netherlands, we visited the home in which our father was born and saw the now-towering tree he had planted as a five-year-old boy eighty-five years earlier. Suddenly, aspects of our cultural background and family history became very significant, perhaps due to the need to understand family events, our age (being in our mid to late 40s), and our need to connect to our Dutch heritage.

PRACTICAL WORKING OR DOING QUALITY

Meaning in life also contains a practical working quality. This practical aspect is often attached to the spiritual and existential component of meaning. When a particular faith, culture, or form of spirituality gives us meaning, we may engage in activities that concretely express meaning, such as attending church services, volunteering for causes that are in line with the tenets of our faith or cultural practices, or contributing monies to charitable organizations. These activities not only reinforce our sense of meaning, but they provide structure to our daily lives and link us with like-minded people (and hence the connection aspect of meaning). The practical working out of meaning can result in a deep sense of doing what one is intended to do in this life, and being involved with something larger than oneself. "I was created to do this!" is one such expression of meaning.

It is important to draw a distinction between meaning derived from faith or spiritual beliefs and meaning gleaned from daily doing. Some individuals in faith communities feel frustrated; yes, they have meaning in regards to having faith that anchors them to the future, such as an afterlife, but meaning in the here and now is somehow absent. They feel reticent to tell others about their feelings of emptiness, for fear that others will tell them they just need to believe or pray more. However, this emptiness does not mean that they lack faith, but perhaps that they need some practical expression of what they believe (Van Tongeren, Green, Davis, Hook, & Hulsey, 2016).

The Relationship Between Meaning and Personal Identity

There is an intricate and reciprocal relationship between meaning and our sense of identity. A sense of meaning defines us as people, and in turn we define what meaning is to us. When our sense of meaning in life is tied to the faith taught to us and fostered in childhood, our identity, in terms of who we are, will be shaped by that faith. We will seek to adapt our ways of thinking and behavior to be in line with the tenets of this faith (for example, following the Golden Rule, in whatever form we have learned it). Sometimes even our choice of profession is shaped by that faith. For instance, we may be drawn to helping professions, such

> There is an intricate and reciprocal relationship between meaning and our sense of identity.

as nursing, education, social work, or the ministry. Or we may look at how we can adapt our skills and talents, such as carpentry, in order to build homes for those who cannot afford home ownership, by volunteering for agencies such as Habitat for Humanity.

Interestingly, however, our identity—how we conceptualize ourselves—also impacts our sense of meaning in life. For instance, when a man views himself as being a good and ethical man, and he values that self-assessment, he will likely derive meaning in continuing to be good and moral and will

> A sense of meaning defines us as people, and in turn we define what meaning is to us.

seek to express those qualities in his work, his leisure activities, and how he relates to others. If he behaves in a way that contradicts this self-assessment (for instance, engaging in an extramarital affair), he will likely experience an identity crisis. "This is not who I am!" he may think. What he does with this contradiction will impact how he sees himself in the future; it will also impact how he views his life in retrospect, as he faces death.

The connection between identity and meaning is often strong when both are tied to a profession. While there is great strength in this—congruency in my values, identity, and work—there is also vulnerability. If I need to leave the profession that is to me a vocation, due to changes in work situation or health, I may feel rocked to the core of my being. Hypothetically, if I am no longer a firefighter who protects the well-being and safety of citizens in my town, who am I? Most likely, the sense of meaning and identity of being a protector of the public is integral to how I see myself, and indeed, view life. Now I have a sense of disequilibrium: I do not know who I am in relation to myself (how do I define myself?), my sense of meaning in life (how am I going to find my value and fill my days?), and how I relate to others (if I cannot serve others by protecting them, what can I do?). Many a retired professional athlete and career military man or woman has struggled terribly in this way, as meaning in life and identity (and, for professional athletes, fame) were tightly tied together, and retirement meant a serious loss of sense of self.

Redefining my sense of significance, or maintaining my sense of meaning but expressing it in another way, may necessitate a difficult and protracted process of grieving, exploration, and transition. Novelist Sue Monk Kidd has referred to this process of "unraveling (my) external identity and coming home to (my) real identity (as) soul work" (Brainy Quote, 2016c). While this work is difficult, if not done, I may flounder in my ability to find purpose in life, to relate to God and others, and to structure my days meaningfully.

This internal work results in a greater sense of meaning in *being*; my worth is not simply in what I can *do*, but also because I *am*. For those who wrest, for those who strive, learning to know and value self for who one *is* can be terrifying. And yet it is tremendously growth-producing. One comes to understand on a deeper level that humanity (and all of creation) has profound value in and of itself; it changes how one views self and the world. Love for others and self, as well as grace for the failings of self and others, are two results. An emphasis in palliative care is providing an atmosphere of love and acceptance: "I've never known such love!" said a dying individual to

Marlette. When he could no longer *do*, but was loved simply because he *was,* it surprised him and gave him the safe space in which to do his end-of-life work.

Our sense of meaning in life often changes over time. For instance, we may find meaning and comfort in childhood in a simple belief system (guided by such axioms as "If I do good, then good will come back to me"). As we grow older, however, and bump up against difficult people and situations, the simple belief that God will reward us if we are good may seem juvenile. An individual may view these beliefs as unscientific, childish, and unsophisticated. The temptation to discard these axioms is reinforced by others who may not be like-minded, or by revered educators or professionals who challenge these ways of thinking.

Interestingly, however, while some individuals discard their childhood faith, they may return to these beliefs in some form or another as they get older and experience pain and loss of control. As decades pass and their sense of control over life wanes, it does not seem so unsophisticated or unscientific to believe that something or Someone has to be in charge; the aging individual realizes that he no longer is capable of being the absolute master of his fate (Lane & Reed, 2015).

Time may also impact how individuals choose to spend their hours and how they perceive life's experiences. For instance, individuals who perceive themselves to have a lot of time left in life spend it "out there"—doing things and relating to those who are not closest to them. But the aged, who know time (and energy) is limited, allocate their twenty-four hours per day to those activities and people who are dearest to them (Fredrickson &

Carstensen, 1998).[2] Also, their experiences can be more poignant, as joy is often mixed with sadness as they anticipate the ending of their lives (Ersner-Hershfield, Mikels, Sullivan, & Carstensen, 2008). More than a century ago, Franz Kafka said that "the meaning of life is that it stops" (Franz Kafka Online, 2016). Without the boundaries of beginnings and endings, it seems that life is not cherished.

The Relationship Between Meaning and Life Events

Life events often have a profound effect upon meaning. For instance, injury or illness may have a tremendous impact upon an individual's sense of meaning. If the injury, such as paralysis due to a car accident, affects an individual's sense of fairness in life, as well as meaning derived from work or providing for his family, then the grief, loss, and anger can be significant.

Depending upon what the individual has learned in his faith or life paradigm, questions about the fairness of God or life may abound. Others, generally well-intended, may inadvertently add to the existential pain of this individual by refusing to listen to his sadness and grief, instead offering platitudes ("God won't give you more than you can handle!"). Particularly if the "comforting" individual inappropriately applies scriptures or theological concepts that do not acknowledge the emotional pain, the newly paralyzed individual will feel like his faith, or those within his faith community, are damning him. This can cause a crisis of faith. The work of finding meaning in

---

2 Interesting, this principle does not just apply to the aged. For much younger people with terminal illness, their limited time is allocated to those people and things that are most important to them. (See Gawande, 2014.)

his accident, as well as meaning in his life, may be a lonely journey. And if this poor man is not able to find some meaning in his life after the accident, he may lose his faith and the support system of his faith group (however weak he found it to be) on top of his mobility—a complex crisis of meaning!

Similarly, a woman who has been defrauded by her business partner and lost a large amount of money has not only taken a financial beating, she may have lost her belief that people are basically good or that if she does good, she will be rewarded. This can be profoundly unsettling and disorienting. This woman, who has prided herself on doing good, may now wonder, "What's the use?" If she cannot trust God, or a business partner she believed was trustworthy, who or what can she trust? She may wonder about her own ability to judge people, making the moving forward after such an event very frightening; her spiritual lenses, if not broken, are deeply scratched.

While time and events can impact our sense of meaning negatively, time with accompanying new experiences can introduce fresh meaning. For instance, some individuals who travel extensively find that their sense of meaning may be expanded as they are exposed to individuals from other parts of the world who hold to very different faiths or beliefs yet act in ways that are in line with their faith or life paradigm. These experiences can be profound in that their beliefs, upon which a sense of meaning rests, may be stretched and changed. In these situations, the change may be unexpected, but growth-producing.

For example, building one's life within a particular faith culture can have advantages: the security of associating with like-minded individuals, built-in social activities through the community, and a shared "language" in understanding life. One may think that his own community has cornered the market on meaning. Interacting with those of other faiths may wonderfully broaden that perception. In one situation, Marlette was dialoguing with a man of another culture and faith. The shared understanding of some of the core principles of life (meaning!) was very apparent, and the conversation was rich. At the end, he said to her, "Sister, the light of God shines from your eyes!" Marlette could echo that statement regarding him, and add a blessing valued by both of their faiths. She will never forget the fellowship, connection, and spirit of that conversation.

BARRIERS TO FINDING AND NURTURING MEANING

Why do some people lack meaning in life? There are a number of reasons. Some individuals are not naturally inclined to look for bigger meaning or purpose in life. They may be engaged in activities that give fun and structure to their lives (e.g. mountain-biking or skiing on the weekends), and this seems to be enough for them, at least in the present. For others, the business and busyness of life leaves little time for the work needed to consider and pursue meaning. Still others may have ardently sought for meaning in the faith system in which they were raised, but they were badly bruised by church leaders in their community. To hold onto this paradigm and the meaning it contains becomes repugnant and even frightening if the behavior of the leaders is not separated in this wounded person's heart and mind from the meaning of faith.

For others, making or nurturing meaning takes too much effort or is too painful. For instance, doing the existential work of asking oneself pertinent questions about life, and one's purpose and direction, may be uncomfortable. It also requires effort and much courage to make decisions to realize the answers to those questions. The one for whom the major question of his later years is "How do I repair my relationship with my son?" will need to take action on his answer. No one else can do that for him. It will demand a lion's heart, it will likely require a plan, and it may take time, but the rewards may be priceless. The fractured relationship (the broken vase) may be restored with seams of gold.

Similarly, wresting meaning from life often requires discipline and sacrifice and may involve pain. The meaning derived from providing education or healthcare to individuals in a developing country can be enormous; however, the discomfort of the heat, the lack of amenities present in developed countries, and the fever and pain that comes from tropical illnesses can be equally enormous. The person who chooses this calling in life understands that the rewards and deep satisfaction of this work is necessarily accompanied by pain. Annette worked as a nurse in a Khmer (Cambodian) refugee camp in 1986–87. The work was hard and the conditions (a hospital comprised of bamboo units, dirt floors, and no running water for the first year) even tougher. Despite this, Annette recognizes how this experience shaped her (and Marlette was glad to get her back in one piece).

A useful and more common analogy is that of parenthood. Parents recognize that the very beings they have brought into this world through the pain of childbirth will also cause them distress through parental concern for their safety and well-being, choices these children make, and the financial sacrifices made to put the kids through school. Much of their work will be done outside of the limelight (if you are a parent, you know this is probably a good thing!). There are no crowds cheering them on; Mother's Day and Father's Day are not sufficient rewards for the energy expended and the difficulties endured. However, the payoff can be enormous in terms of the intangibles of purpose in life, meaning ("That's my daughter up there, receiving her diploma!"), and the joy of seeing them grow into productive adults.

Another barrier to finding meaning in life in western societies is the emphasis on independence and autonomy. The close ties to family that were part and parcel of life one hundred years ago have been significantly weakened through geographic mobility; families that lived for generations in one area are now spread all over the world. The meaning gleaned from helping family members, particularly aged ones, is lost to our focus on being self-sufficient and autonomous. Relatedly, the focus in the media and in our approach to living tends towards the self: self-esteem, self-actualization, even "selfies". This type of orientation promotes self-expression and development, perhaps giving individuals more freedom (a son does not necessarily have to take on his father's business, for example). However, the roots to the past can be weakened; the foundation stones of identity can be buried.

In addition to an emphasis on independence and autonomy, western society could also be described as hedonistic, or pleasure-seeking. Fun and instant happiness achieved through movies, television, and video games seem more enticing than the hard-fought gains of meaning. Thus, young people may live with their parents, choosing to work part-time to allow them to pursue personal interests well into their thirties. Rather than launching in their early twenties, the responsibilities (and rewards) of adulthood are delayed, with fun being the primary goal. Ironically, "it is the very pursuit of happiness that thwarts happiness" (Viktor Frankl, Goodreads, 2016b). Recent thought corroborates this (Furnham, 2014; Kashdan, 2010). As Furnham (2014) stated, "(Happiness) is like soap in the bath. The more you try to grab it, the more cloudy the water: the more difficult it is to find."

In 2000, psychologists Daniel Gilbert and Timothy Wilson coined the word *miswanting* (and its subsequent derivatives: miswants, miswanted, etc.). To miswant is to mistakenly believe that something acquired—a new car or home renovations—will make one happy. Initially, there may be pleasure, but that new acquisition will soon become the norm, and pleasure will be lost. The consumer focus of North America, promising happiness if the lottery is won or the trip is realized, contributes to miswanting; the pursuit of happiness ironically thwarts its realization.

The pursuit of meaning in day-to-day life, as well as the larger-than-life situations we encounter, guarantees wresting, but it also assures value and worth in living; indeed, it may well produce happiness as a byproduct of the existential work. John Dewey says, "Such happiness as life is capable of comes from the full participation of all our powers in the endeavor to wrest from each changing situation of experience its own full and unique meaning" (Thinkexist.com, 2016).

And, sadly, some situations in this life are just plain grueling; finding meaning in them can be excruciating. Caring for a spouse sliding into the vortex of dementia is soul-wrenching. The very demands of twenty-four-hour caregiving can work against any sense of personal growth when one is simply attempting to make it from day to day. Is there meaning in the suffering for both the spouse with dementia and the caregiver? We believe so. Towards the end of the book, we will discuss the soul work of older adulthood—looking within so that one does not simply cope, but thrives with the challenges of their last years.

We started this chapter with the famous quote from the writer of the book of Ecclesiastes. Depending upon the version of the book, he felt that life was useless, meaningless, pointless, vanity. The Bible does not sugar-coat human experience; it is expressed in all its glory and ugliness. And it could be safely said that the author of this biblical book was not writing from a position of emotional health! Schwartz (Goodreads, 2016a) also spoke of many North Americans living in ways that are meaningless. These statements do not mean that there is not meaning to be had, but rather that meaning has to be cultivated, mined, sought after, and worked for. It is made, not bestowed upon. More on how to do this as we continue.

QUESTIONS TO PONDER:
- What gives you meaning in life? How has this changed as you age, or as you observe loved ones age?
- How does your life paradigm influence your sense of meaning?

- Upon reflection, do you find yourself miswanting? What is the focus of your miswants?
- What impact does faith have upon your day-to-day living? Do your beliefs have practical expressions that bring meaning to you, and to others?

TIPS FOR CONSIDERATION:
- Take thirty minutes to write down how you spend your free time. Consider how your free activities coincide with what gives you meaning in life.
- Based upon the evaluation of activities and their relationship to meaning in your life, what activities will you change? What activities will you keep?

chapter two

WHY MEANING IS SO IMPORTANT IN AGING

And the King will answer them, "Truly, I say to you, as you did it to one of the least of these my brethren, you did it to me."
—Matthew 25:40 (RSV)

A nation's greatness is measured by how it treats its weakest members.
—Mahatma Gandhi
leader in the struggle for Indian independence
(topix.com, 2016)

In this book, we contend that making meaning in life is very important for all individuals, but it's particularly critical for older adults. Why would the well-being of any particular group be so vital to the whole? We start this chapter examining why meaning is so important to older adults. We then consider the importance of meaning within the aging family, and then broadly, throughout society as a whole. In all of this, we wish to assert that *society needs older adults as much as older adults need society.*

Annette M. Lane and Marlette B. Reed

OLDER ADULTS AND MEANING

Certainly, experiencing meaning in life is valuable at any age. However, we argue that for older adults, finding and fostering meaning is critical. Unfortunately, the significance of meaning in aging is often not recognized. Within this section, we will examine how societal values impact older adults' sense of identity, as well as how life experiences such as retirement and health changes as well as dying and death can influence how aging individuals conceptualize their lives and worth.

SOCIETAL VALUES

Much has been said about western society's orientation toward youth. Adolescents and young adults are lauded as being beautiful, intelligent, productive, and possessing great potential and opportunities. While celebrating youth and young adulthood as rich and fruitful times is not inherently wrong, we ask, how does this value system impact aging adults, and how accurate are these values?

The major emphasis on physical beauty, which is conceptualized as youthful skin (lacking facial wrinkles and age spots), is everywhere in the media. With this has come a burgeoning acceptance of plastic surgery to assist older adults to look younger. No longer relegated to a few women who subject themselves to facelifts, procedures such as injections and implants make attaining a youthful appearance more available to men and women, and as availability and acceptability have grown, sometimes these procedures have become almost necessary for one's career and social viability (Honigman & Castle, 2006).

Aging is understood to be "a pathological condition in need of correction or repair; a 'disease', which modern medicine must combat" (Honigman & Castle, 2006, np).

With more and more aging adults utilizing youth-enhancing procedures, a subtle yet significant shift has occurred in society as a whole. Why should aging individuals look old when they don't have to?[3] And if one does not have to look a certain way that is understood to represent old age, the implicit message is that older age is not valued. If aging is not valued, then neither are older adults valued. Aging and its telltale signs become feared, resulting in older individuals paying large sums of money and exerting great effort to look younger. While plastic surgery and procedures to look younger are individual decisions, we oppose the underlying assumptions that youthfulness is better than aging, and that older adults are less valuable members of society than the young.

RETIREMENT OR JOB LOSS

While some aging adults greatly look forward to retirement, others dread this time of life. Not only has work encapsulated their identities, but it has provided structure and purpose to their days. In later years, when they no longer go to a job or perform specific duties, they see their lives as less than what they were in the past. Their working years (whether within or outside the home) were the years when they felt most productive; they felt like they were giving. "There's not much left here for me," said

---

3 Nora Ephron rails against the trends that push aging women to look a decade (or more) younger than their chronological age. Wryly she states, "Sometimes I think that not having to worry about your hair anymore is the secret upside of death." (Ephron, 2008, 32).

our mother after her kids were raised and on their own. While many older adults are able to reinvent themselves through new passions and roles, our mother never really was. Her children's best efforts at getting her involved in other things did not lead to a successful transition. Sadly, in many ways, life became meaningless for her.

Finding meaning becomes particularly pertinent at this point in life. Through daily work, adults have been able to derive a sense of meaning, or have delayed facing the lack of meaning in their lives. Upon retirement, they are either starkly challenged with having lost their sense of meaning or confronted with their need to find it. And while there may be enticing opportunities out there, some of these older adults lack the financial means to realize them. As the familiar saying goes, "Retirement can be a great joy if you can figure out how to spend time without spending money" (Author unknown, Quote Garden, 2016a). With these challenges, some aging adults rise to the occasion and find this time of life satisfying and even growth-producing, while some quell their soul unrest with self-medication in the form of substances; others languish in despair.

HEALTH CHANGES

Older adults experience health changes related to normal aging (such as changes in vision or sleep patterns) as well as changes like chronic pain, arthritis, and diabetes. Chronic pain and changes in functional abilities (what a person can and cannot do) can have a profound effect on how older adults conceptualize themselves and their abilities, especially when they cannot engage in activities they have found enjoyable or meaningful. If older adults find that life no longer affords them the enjoyment they once experienced, they may wonder, as our mother did, what is left for them. Finding activities that can engage these older adults meaningfully, even though they have lost some physical capabilities, becomes much more critical than when they were younger and had full functional abilities. Increasingly, meaning is found to be an important aspect of health and well-being, even in environments such as nursing homes (Haugan, 2014b). Having meaning contributes to physical and mental health.

DYING AND DEATH

Aging adults often refer to the number of funerals they attend of acquaintances, friends, and family members. They relate the emotional toll it takes upon them to see their contemporaries, and even individuals younger than them, pass away. They may feel tempted to just sit (physically and metaphorically) and wait for death to take them. We can certainly understand this and would never want to minimize the profound grief experienced with the deaths of spouses, family members, or friends. However, we suggest that maintaining meaning in life, or discovering new meaning, is critical to the ability of widows and widowers to deal with death's challenges. In Chapter Four, we will discuss the meaning that can come from heading into dying and death.

CHRONIC SORROW

Kaethe Weingarten (2012) discussed the topic of chronic sorrow. She addressed this construct as something an individual feels when her body physically does not represent how she sees herself. This woman's body is not what it used to be due to progressive illness or expected deterioration tied to injury (the long-term complications of paralysis, for example); with this can also come the haunting question: what will this body be like in the future? The losses are expected to mount, and in this an individual can experience profound, ongoing sorrow. She is not able to express herself in ways that are congruent with her self-conceptualization (Weingarten, 2012). For instance, this woman may view herself as an athlete who can no longer participate in activities that reinforced her identity. The loss is much greater than the activities themselves; the loss also entails how she views herself and portrays herself to others. And as further deterioration may occur in the future, the self, in whatever form the deterioration takes, may seem tenuous.

Older adults may experience chronic sorrow in relation to changes in health, the loss of activities that defined them, and a loss of identity. Chronic sorrow may greatly impact how they view their lives and their futures. Often, however, this sorrow may be insidious, whereby aging adults don't recognize this as something they need to address or combat. They may even be lulled into the sense that this continuous sorrow is "normal" in aging. While we admit that facing into changes that occur with aging can be difficult, we suggest that meaning can be an antidote. If individuals have a strong sense of meaning and can sustain that (through creative avenues), they will be more likely to recognize the chronic sorrow, with its fear and potential hopelessness, and combat it with courage and purpose (Haugan, 2014a).

OLDER ADULTS, MEANING, AND THE INFLUENCE UPON THE FAMILY

When aging adults feel and demonstrate despair and significant existential angst, family members, such as adult children and grandchildren, notice. Adult children may express frustration over an aging parent not being able to cope with life and inadvertently share their irritation and disappointment with their own children. Deep down, however, adult children may wonder, "Is this what my life will come to?" They may genuinely fear aging. Their aging parents may have no idea how much their family members are watching and the lessons they are learning from them.

Relatedly, these aging adults may not realize how crucial their example is to their children and grandchildren. Aging adults who remain engaged in life, and communicate to their family members what they are doing and their excitement in following these passions, reveal to their family members that life can be meaningful, full of purpose, and worthwhile, even at an advanced age.

We had an uncle who lived in the Netherlands. Almost yearly, Uncle Jan would travel to Canada to visit his sisters. Our father would often take our uncle out for dinner; our dad loved to see Jan, as he was deeply engaged in life and could intelligently discuss politics and ideas! When he died at ninety-two years of age, we felt sad. Our sadness was not due to a sense that Uncle Jan's life was meaningless in his latter years (it wasn't), but rather that his life seemed cut short when he died, as he was so young at heart and engaged in living!

Annette M. Lane and Marlette B. Reed

Older Adults, Meaning, and Society

Some cultures revere their elders more than others. Traditionally, Asian cultures have respected and honored older adults more than western cultures. When elderly individuals lived with their children until death, they fulfilled a significant role in the family. They were respected for their years, wisdom, and knowledge. They interacted daily with their children and grandchildren; *their lives and experiences taught their family members how to face advancing age and death.* This is changing as some Asian countries, such as India, adopt North American values.

Multigenerational Families

Multigenerational families, once customary, are becoming less common in Asian countries such as India. With multigenerational living arrangements less frequent than decades ago, the nuclear family has emerged, and is considered typical of urban living. In a 2012 report, the International Longevity Centre Global Alliance indicated that in Indian cities, less than thirty percent of the homes are "joint families," although they are more common in rural areas, where the percentage of multigenerational households is still more than sixty percent (Raje, 2012). This social trend away from multigenerational living arrangements is expected to continue, as working age Indians move from rural homes to the cities to work and as western norms are adopted.

In North America, relatively few older adults live with their adult children. A Pew Research Center study (2014) indicated that in the U.S. in 2012, only 18.1 percent of American households were multigenerational.

Further, a 2012 Gallup and Robinson study indicated that while fifty-one percent of adult children would be willing to have a parent who could no longer live on their own join their household, only thirty-one percent of older adults would consider doing so (Bradley Bursack, 2015).

Without living in close proximity, adult children and grandchildren globally are less likely to hear the stories of the aged adult and learn from his/her experiences. They are less likely to receive advice from this individual; even though the aged parent may still see family members, opportunities to impart wisdom and maintain their respected place in the family may be infrequent and diminished.

DEMOGRAPHIC DIVIDE

Whether the result of societal emphasis upon the young, or from the effects of the Industrial Revolution (with its emphasis upon productivity and efficiency), there is a significant demographic divide between the young and the old. Education is a form of mass production, where children are grouped according to age (and sometimes, within the age groupings, according to ability). Older adults and youth are usually separated in faith communities as well.

We offer seminars in churches about issues of aging, and one lovely older woman spoke with us following a session. She remarked that older adults were always kept apart from the youth and how enjoyable it would be to have the occasional get-together with youth. We heartily agreed! Generations need to intermingle within communities. Through interactions while playing board games, for example, youth could discover how fun aging persons can be, and aging adults could recognize how amusing the youth are. Relationships could be developed so that when the youth and aged pass each other when entering or leaving church, they could interact freely. Friendships could be forged and youth could develop a sense of what it is like for individuals to age, both the challenges and joys. Through relationship with aging adults, youth may learn that aging is not to be feared and that life can be meaningful and fulfilling in later decades.

How Should Aging Adults Respond?

As challenging as aging can be, particularly within the context of a youth-oriented society, older adults can actively respond. By purposefully responding, older adults tend to their needs for meaning but also illustrate to a youth-oriented society that aging can involve fulfillment.

Contributions to Society

We firmly believe that older adults need to actively look for areas in which they can contribute to society. They need to consider what is meaningful to them (see Chapter Five regarding a mini life review) rather than just filling an organization's needs.

For instance, in the past, an aging individual might have stuffed envelopes for a not-for-profit agency when said agency was blitzing its membership or donors. Even though there was and is nothing wrong with this activity, and certainly someone needs to complete the non-glamorous tasks, we believe that aging adults should consider their strengths and goals for the future, and choose activities that enhance their sense of meaning.

Certainly, they can contribute time and physical labor (e.g. stocking shelves at a food bank), but they also can contribute the experience of their years and their ability to relate—to connect—with others. They bring resilience (with "tools in the toolbox" for dealing with problems) and respect for reciprocity (while they have experience to offer an organization, they can benefit from that organization too).

Marlette worked as a chaplain in a hospice for a number of years; some of the most effective volunteers with the residents were older adults who had experienced life and death. Their ability to relate to dying residents and their families was exquisite. Watching older adults with doctoral degrees tenderly feed a dying resident breakfast or read poetry to her never ceased to move Marlette deeply. It was truly a spiritual experience to watch people *connect* with people.

And older volunteers bring years of professional know-how to whatever they involve themselves in. The knowledge and wisdom they can impart to those working in agencies is invaluable. With many companies employing contractors or young people, the wisdom of what works and what does not is often missing. Thus, companies may make the same errors they did years earlier, as staff are too young (chronologically or in years of service) to foresee the problems that will arise with specific decisions or directions. Aging adults can advise with wisdom; they can offer examples of why something did not work and how such mistakes can be avoided.

Aging adults may wonder how meaningful of a contribution can be made in older life. While we recognize that the example of former United States President Jimmy Carter may seem out of the ordinary and not applicable to everyone, Carter is well-regarded for his work after the presidency, with much of this work occurring in older age. Not only have he and his wife been very active with Habitat for Humanity, Carter has been active in world affairs, written many books, and received a Nobel Peace Prize in 2002. Certainly, his aging years have not been meaningless.

Carter's example may not be applicable to most of us. However, the following may be more relevant. In an interesting article by Verena Menec (Evidence Network, 2012), she combatted the notion of the grey tsunami being catastrophic and outlined the contributions of older adults. In addition to volunteering and paying taxes, Menec noted that aging adults are substantial givers and allocate more donations to charity than any other age groups. Further, Menec tied their family work, such as caring for grandchildren, an ailing spouse, or other aging adults in the community, to the economy. By virtue of providing care to grandchildren, women with children can work outside the home, and by giving care to an ailing wife or neighbor, there are less demands upon the health care system than otherwise would be; thus, by their actions, the economy is benefitted and the drains on the health care system are lessened (Evidence Network, 2012). On a broader scale, while acknowledging the challenges of global aging, the United Nations said that aging "is a triumph of development" (UNPF, 2012, p. 16).

ADVOCATING FOR INTERGENERATIONAL ACTIVITIES

In relation to participation in churches, community centers, or other kinds of clubs, older adults can advocate for joint activities with youth, such as meals where youth and older adults are interspersed at tables (to ensure that youth do not congregate at several tables and older adults at others), game evenings, movie nights, and so on. The importance of developing relationships goes far beyond the "niceness" of such ideas. What older adults can teach youth, just in being who they are and sharing their lives, is vital to the development of youth! And conversely, youth can teach older adults what it is to be interested in life and relationships; this may help aging adults remain actively engaged in life, relationships, and ideas. Older adults who have grandchildren across the country (or the world) have the opportunity to grandparent, to some degree, a few young people—and younger people with grandparents far away then have surrogate grandparents close at hand. It's a win-win situation!

These ideas are not new. Certainly, there are programs in the U.S. that purposefully place youth and aging individuals together.[4] In Canada, there is at least one Christian camp that pairs grandparents with needy kids, one to one; here an elder with much to give becomes the buddy of this child for the week at camp. We suggest that older adults should consciously consider what gives them meaning and what causes are important to them and get involved. Further, if they attend church, they can advocate for activities which combine youth and older adults.

These ideas may be encapsulated in the concept of self-transcendence. Self-transcendence refers to a

---

4 We write about this in another book. See Lane and Reed, 2015 in the reference list.

process of maturing—a gradual shift—whereby adults, as they move into older age, experience

the expansion of one's conceptual boundaries inwardly through introspective activities, outwardly through concerns about others' welfare, temporally by integrating perceptions of one's past and future to enhance the present. (Reed, 1991, p. 71)

The older adult looks inward (beliefs and private expressions of the soul, such as journaling), looks outward towards the needs of others, and looks at the past and the future (things hoped for) to infuse the present with meaning. The beauty of understanding self-transcendence is that aging adults can look for and find meaning through various avenues. If an older woman finds herself less able to volunteer, she may continue her inward and outward expansion of boundaries through knitting blankets. She may knit a number of blankets and have a loved one bring them to a homeless shelter. She is thus expressing her inward beliefs about helping others outwardly through knitting (expressing creativity) and giving to others who are less fortunate (altruism).

This same woman can expand her inner boundaries through spiritual practices, such as meditation, prayer, and contemplation. She can bring congruity between the past and present by reflecting upon her life. If she suffered a wound in her past that left her with angst, perhaps even bitterness, she can bring present understanding of the frailty of life (which often becomes clearer as one gets older) to that past interpersonal conflict. She may realize that the person who hurt her did not have the capacity to handle that conflict (he lacked the tools in the toolbox) and can feel a certain pity for this individual—a concept known as deferred empathy (Gunther, 2008). In that place of understanding, this individual may extend, within herself, forgiveness to the one who hurt her. Weaving together this new understanding with her old hurt can bring a rich, beautiful depth to the tapestry of her life. This may not lead to a reestablishment of relationship (and indeed, it can be unwise to reestablish relationship if that connection would be unsafe), but it can lead to greater internal freedom—an expansion of the inner boundaries—of this woman. As well, her hope in heaven brings meaning to the present as she realizes that the way she handles the challenges of each day, and how she deals with outstanding issues from her past, are relevant to others and to the Other. In all of these ways, this dear lady is self-transcending—expanding her connection with God, others, and herself (Haugan, Rannestad, Hammervold, Garasen, & Espnes, 2013)—as the external world for her becomes limited.

Despite the emphasis upon youth and youthfulness, our society needs older people as much as they need society. The aged model what it is to age well; they provide wisdom to younger generations, and connection with so many. They are an invaluable part of the paid and unpaid workforce, and

> Society needs older adults as much as older adults need society.

the economy. And by their very presence, they draw from others what we, as a society, need so badly: to keep living sane and safe.

QUESTIONS TO PONDER:

- What aspects of aging in a youth-oriented society do you find most difficult?
- If you are older, what kind of contact do you have with youth, and what kind of contact would you like to have?

TIPS FOR CONSIDERATION:

- If you belong to a faith community or community center, how can you integrate the youth and aging members for one or more activities?
- What would that activity entail? How would you engage both youth and aging members in the planning and operationalization of the activity?

chapter three

Finding Meaning in the Mundane

But in the end, does it really make a difference what anyone does?

...I've decided that there's nothing better to do than go ahead and have a good time and get the most we can out of life. That's it—eat, drink, and make the most of your job. It's God's gift.

—Ecclesiastes 3:9, 12–13 (The Message)

Creativity is piercing the mundane to find the marvelous.

—Bill Moyers
American journalist and political commentator
(Brainy Quotes, 2016d)

*M*undane is not a terrible word or horrible state, and yet it is often assigned this connotation. Within the western thrill-seeking culture, the notion of the mundane seems antithetical to excitement. The mundane becomes associated with boredom rather than a necessary and even meaningful part of our existence. How in the world can the mundane in life be meaningful? In this chapter, we consider the definition of mundane. We then address how the ordinary is critical to our lives as human beings, and how the mundane, although often viewed as boring, can yield genuine meaning.

DEFINITION OF MUNDANE

According to the Free Online Dictionary (2016), there are two aspects to the concept of mundane: 1) "of, relating to, or typical of this world; secular" and 2) "relating to, characteristic of, or concerned with commonplaces; ordinary." We believe that both aspects of the mundane can be considered when finding meaning.

First, the mundane refers to the material world. It involves the everyday activities of living that ground us in this world—the here and now. There often seems to be a grinding quality to these activities. Laundry has to be done weekly, and no matter how many loads are dumped into the washer and dryer, more laundry always needs to be done. Cleaning the house is regularly done, yet somehow the house always gets dirty again and needs further cleaning. The unending quality to this work seems tiring and not at all connected to meaning. However, we believe that it is. Why?

Day-to-day activities that have to be completed, no matter how mind-numbing, provide structure to our lives. Structure often provides profound yet unrecognized meaning in this world. That is, until that structure is gone.

An example may be helpful. Bob, a sixty-year-old man, worked in the business world for years and now is off work due to an injury and is receiving disability benefits. He finds himself feeling strangely off-kilter. When he was working, he often became tired of getting up early each weekday morning, driving to work, toiling a full day with some people he liked, and others, well, not so much. Then, as Bob drove home in rush-hour traffic, he often felt frustrated by the gridlock on busy thoroughfares; he passed the time mulling over the day's events, sometimes fuming as he remembered the odd unpleasant interaction. When he arrived home, he would sit for dinner with Jean, his spouse, watch the news on TV, then doze on the couch before collapsing into bed. Now, on disability, Bob honestly wonders why he feels so adrift; after all, he had become tired of this aforementioned routine.

Yet that routine and structure gave purpose to Bob's day, even if that structure was largely dictated by others. It also facilitated interaction with others; those exchanges provided a sense of not being alone in this often lonely world. It also provided conversation with others about interesting ideas and goings-on in their families, which became a springboard for conversation with Jean in the evening. The structure also facilitated a sense of accomplishment. At the end of the day, Bob could ponder what he had done and still needed to do. As part of this sense of accomplishment, Bob was learning new skills and ideas in his work, which provided a sense of vitality. Even though this structure was grounded in the day-to-day, it also enabled learning and allowed him to look forward to future projects. At the end of a workweek, the lack of structure became a delicious reward for his labor.

Everyday life had meaning and purpose and future-oriented thinking, even if it was stressful. Now, Bob finds himself wandering around his home, turning his TV on and off, playing computer games, and, overall, feeling aimless and lost. He now realizes that there was deeper meaning to his daily work life that he never recognized or appreciated. Bob is sad; he's always seen himself as the family provider. This was a key part of his identity. Now, with his injury, he's not sure he'll ever work again (the insidious onset of chronic sorrow perhaps). Bob also wonders and worries about how his life will unfold in the future; how will he make something new of his life when work, as he once knew it, no longer exists?

The second part of the definition of mundane refers to commonplace or ordinary activities. These activities were described in Bob's story. The link of these activities to finding meaning was explained in terms of the connection of structure to meaning. It also perhaps hinted that this structure may lead to interactions with others. What it did not do is illuminate the quality of those interactions. For instance, in the past when Bob went home and talked with Jean over dinner about his day, he may have expressed great concern about a colleague at work who was going through a difficult divorce. As Jean listened to her spouse, her heart may have felt compassion for this colleague of Bob; she also may have felt pride and love for the character of her husband. Through the ordinary, mundane activity of talking to a colleague at work, Bob became aware of a deep need. Then he and Jean, united in their concern, came up with a plan to support him through his difficult time. Through this collaboration on a plan and carrying it out, Bob and Jean felt a sense of greater meaning in their daily lives. And though there were stressful interactions at work, by far the majority of these connections were not, and some were even life-giving, affirming; it has taken this time on disability for Bob to clean his spiritual lenses and see that.

Continuing with Bob and Jean's story and the importance of the mundane in their lives, one ordinary activity that has been part of their regular routine involves babysitting their eight-year-old grandson several evenings a week while his mom works the late shift. Bob has always played physically with young Jake, who does not have a dad in his life and seems to need to roughhouse. Bob and Jean have sometimes grown tired of this routine. After all, they have raised their kids; aren't they too old for this? And yet now that Bob is home, and no longer able to play as roughly, he misses these interactions. But they are outward-focused enough to see Jake's care for his poppa. Their hearts are touched and moved by their grandson's gentle and respectful love which briefly, albeit imperfectly, speaks to them of God's gentle and tender love. Their ordinary activity of regular Jake time reminds them of God's image stamped upon humanity—in particular, their grandson. The mundane, that which is of this world and ordinary, connects them to that which is transcendent.

THE IMPORTANCE OF THE MUNDANE TO EVERYDAY LIFE

The mundane—the ordinary routine of daily life—is critical to our existence as human beings. The first part of the definition indicates "typical of this world" (Free Online Dictionary, 2016). What could be more typical than soil, than dirt? Humus, the result of decaying plant matter, such as leaves, is a part of soil. And in Latin, humus means earth (soil). The word *human* is often connected

> The mundane – the ordinary routine of daily life – is critical to our existence as human beings.

with this, the thought being that humanity came from the ground (the creation story). Our humanity is predicated upon being "typical of this world." In past centuries, when economies were primarily agrarian, humans literally worked daily for their living with the soil of the earth. They were literally connected to the land. Humans and humus: of this world, earthy, ordinary, mundane.

Today, the everyday routines of living are often not carried out in or with the soil of the earth. They involve chores around the house, as well as the tasks we complete for loved ones, and these routines provide structure to our lives and create a rhythm that gives us security. If we were to complete new chores every day, our lives would be in constant chaos. We would not be able to do the business of living. The stress of having to learn new things daily would mean that we would accomplish less, and experience far more mental and physical pressure. Our survival might be in jeopardy!

The truth of one's need for routine is evident in those experiencing dementia. Sadly, dementia robs individuals of the abilities to conduct everyday tasks such as getting dressed, brushing teeth, and preparing a meal. Particularly as the dementia progresses, affected individuals can accomplish very little without help; they simply are not able to figure out how to do simple tasks. These problems, however, are exacerbated even more when those with dementia are removed from their environments to go on a trip, or when changing living locations.

Another example may be useful. Those who are homeless cannot accomplish what most of us would consider normal tasks of daily living. They cannot prepare a meal for themselves as they are on the streets and do not have access to a stove and groceries. They cannot wash and bathe like those living in their own homes, as they do not have regular access to showers. Their days are relegated to finding a place to sleep for the night (perhaps at a shelter), finding some form of sustenance (at a soup kitchen, collecting bottles, panhandling) and being on the lookout for dangers. The routines that give structure to our lives, but also make our daily living easier so that we can accomplish more, are not available to those on the streets. Clearly, having routines and life circumstances that sustain routines (such as intact cognition, homes, work) are critical to daily functioning.

THE ADDED IMPORTANCE OF THE MUNDANE AS WE AGE: NOURISHING OUR SOULS

We suggest that the mundane, while always important, becomes more important as we age. There are several reasons for this. The mundane provides structure and activities that we need to engage in. The mundane brings us into contact with others. Even when we do not seek out that contact, the ordinary extracts creativity out of us if we choose to find meaning in it. And finally, the mundane invites us to find beauty in nature and what we see.

PROVISION OF STRUCTURE

First, routines and the structure/activities they provide force us to be active, at least to some degree. Meals need to be cooked, housework done, and laundry washed. These activities provide some rationale for getting out of bed in the morning. The physical act of moving as we age becomes more important; those who regularly move physically do better than those who do not. For the many older adults concerned about fitness, doing those loads of laundry—perhaps not meaningful in and of itself—can contribute to the distance they wish to walk in a day. When tasks have to be done, older adults get up to do them, and even if they find themselves lacking motivation, the motivation often comes after several tasks are completed and a lovely sense of accomplishment washes over them.

Interestingly, the reverse can be true. In some countries where the cost of living is high, adults in their thirties or forties may return to the home of their aging parents after experiencing a loss of job or a divorce. Sometimes, these adults do little because they are upset or depressed over their life circumstances. They may lie in bed until the early afternoon, walk around the house in an unkempt state, and then stay up late playing computer games and watching television. Their aging parents may feel befuddled as to how their adult children can be so aimless and unmotivated. However, doing nothing often begets doing nothing. When we are forced to do what needs to be done in terms of household tasks and the activities of daily living, we often are better off physically and mentally; in this way, the soul is nourished.

CONTACT WITH OTHERS

Engaging in daily routines connects us with others, even when we don't naturally seek others out. By virtue of having to pick up a few groceries, we may talk with someone waiting in line behind us at the till. Then, when we pay for our groceries, the cashier may inquire how we are doing. This contact is facilitated by the mundane of life.

We remember that a few days after our mother died, we took our father out for dinner. Then we needed to stop by the pharmacy to drop off our mother's leftover medications for disposal. The routine activity of visiting the pharmacist provided the opportunity for the pharmacist to express his sincere condolences to our father and give him a card. Not only was our father touched by this expression of concern, the mundane activity of regularly talking with the pharmacist over a period of years allowed meaningful contact for Dad in his mourning; in those dark days after our mother's death, his soul was nourished.

Walking a dog can also facilitate wonderful contact with others. Recent Canadian research reveals that older adults who walk dogs are more likely to feel positively about their neighborhoods than those who walk without a pet (Toohey, McCormack, Doyle-Baker, Adams, & Rock, 2013). And those who do not have a pet are more likely to feel safe interacting with a dog-walker than a person without a pet (White, 2016). Hence, a dog becomes a vehicle of communication between two individuals passing each other when walking in the opposite direction. The individual who is approaching you sees your dog, and then may stop to ask questions about your dog or to ask if she can pet him. This often becomes the springboard through which the unknown person can talk about her pet or a pet that has passed. There can be an honest understanding between pet owners as they relate stories about the personalities of their pets and the roles they play in the family home. For some, particularly those who have been hurt by others, pets can seem more loyal and reliable than the people in their lives. Exchanging stories about a beloved pet can allow for *meaningful contact with people*; even though they may not seek meaningful contact with others, that meaty connection with others is still important.

EXACTING CREATIVITY

By its very nature, the mundane can be boring. Activities that have been performed so many times over so many years are often completed almost without conscious thought. Thus, wresting meaning out of the mundane demands creativity. Can you engage in the same activities in different ways? For instance, if you walk regularly but are tired of walking alone in your neighborhood, would you consider walking with others at a nearby mall? Not only will this change your routine, it may facilitate connections or friendships with others who you otherwise would not have met. If you used to bake for family members—and indeed, were considered a master of pastry—but have given up baking because you live alone, could you begin baking again, not just for yourself but for others you know in your community or church? Giving the products to others becomes about much more than the physical act of baking; it becomes the means through which you can share your talents with others and truly bless them. You may find that you give a pie to someone who is intensely lonely and feels invisible, even unloved. Your gift may encourage her that she is not alone and create the context whereby she feels comfortable talking with you. She may share her loneliness that developed when her spouse passed away, and this may become a catalyst for regular telephone conversations and occasional coffee dates.

Through the act of baking and gifting that baking to another in need, you may experience the beauty of this suffering individual, help her by your presence and wisdom, and be in turn helped because you have found an outlet for that which is in you to give. The creativity that was exacted from you has led to a soul-nourishing opportunity and relationship.

MOVEMENT IN THE MUNDANE

We often do not realize the exquisite joy of movement; after all, we have been moving since birth. But as we age and experience bodily changes, such as arthritis or chronic pain, movement may become painful; movement without discomfort may be then experienced as a gift, not a given. Moreover, if we consider how we can move our bodies through time and space, the ability to move can be delightful. Occasionally, we will swim in a neighborhood lake during the summer. As the lake is cold, we tend to swim only in very hot weather. As we swim the perimeter of the lake (once we have withstood the shock of the cold water!), there is a sense of genuine pleasure to move our bodies through the water (the medium) across time (the hour that we swim). Not only do we experience the sense of accomplishment as we tabulate how far we have swum, but we have the palpable sensation of the warm sun on our faces, the visual beauty of the sun reflecting off the waves (creating diamonds on the crests), and the sounds of children screaming and yelling with delight. Marlette has rheumatoid arthritis, and in the cold water this extensive effort is easier than exertion on land; she never ceases to appreciate how wonderful it is to stretch her muscles and her limits!

Continuing to move as we age is extremely important and can be meaningful. To keep on moving in spite of disabilities impacts our physical and mental health in positive ways. When working out at community gyms, we have sometimes witnessed older men or women who exercise despite having suffered a stroke. (We recognize the signs of a previous stroke, as there is pronounced one-sided bodily weakness.) We don't know whether to cry, out of empathy, or laugh and clap in delight for the sheer guts and determination they exhibit! Truly, *we are moved by their movement.* These courageous individuals may find meaning in their movement as they emphasize to themselves their abilities (rather than disabilities), interact with others in the gym, and experience the satisfaction that comes with exercise. While we caution that older adults should seek the advice of their physician regarding the types of exercise that are appropriate for them, movement is part of meaning in the mundane of life; it feeds the soul.

BEAUTY IN THE MUNDANE

Most people would quickly assert that nature—the blue sky, mountains, lakes, grass, and trees—is beautiful. Some would state that the stark eeriness of the desert is gorgeous; in particular, they point to the exquisite beauty of desert flowers juxtaposed with the desolation of seeming barrenness. Commonly, however, many do not pay attention to nature in daily life. The cares and concerns of relationships, work, and life dominate their thinking. When life stands still—for example, when a man receives a cancer diagnosis—suddenly he recognizes the colors of autumn leaves. The leaves are not just turning colors; they are *brilliant* reds, *vibrant* yellows, and *jazzy* oranges. And the reds, oranges and yellows are not identical; there are interesting variations within each of these colors. The leaves that have fallen are not just dead, their decomposition into the soil (humus) emits a rich, earthy smell that is accentuated by the warmth of the afternoon fall air. The odor powerfully evokes memories of when this man walked home from school, uproariously laughing as he and his friends purposefully shuffled their feet through the dead leaves to hear the delightful crunches and crackles.

It is tragic that we often do not realize the exquisite beauty in nature until an event or diagnosis changes our focus.[5] If we regularly seek to truly experience nature as we walk, including feeling the quality of the air, hearing the birds chirp and sing, and looking at the spring buds on the trees as they slowly, over the course of weeks, emerge into a fresh flush of green, we will find ourselves less bored and more engaged. We may feel part of something much greater than ourselves and thus enhance the sense of meaning in our lives; our souls—not just our lungs— may be nourished, tended, and nurtured as we breathe in deeply the spring air. We may even purchase a book on trees to understand the types of trees in our neighborhood or nearby parks; this book may become a source of interest when we are at home. Perhaps we will take pictures of the spring daffodils as they begin to open, and keep loved ones across the continent up to date on the progress of spring through regular pictures attached to emails or text

---

5 As mentioned earlier, an awareness of the brevity of life often creates an appreciation for all it contains, even (and sometimes particularly) things previously overlooked.

messages. Connection—to nature, to activities imbued with meaning, to others—brings meaning to the mundane.

In an interesting study of the meaning in life among the oldest of old, Jonsen, Norberg and Lundmen (2014) interviewed three men and seven women between the ages of eighty-five to ninety-five. These individuals talked about the connection of nature to meaning; memories of working in nature were part of what gave their lives meaning (Jonsen et al., 2014). Present-day experiences with nature evoked precious memories from the past, integrating the present with the past (part of self-transcendence), tending, and nourishing the soil of their souls. As such, nature is not just meaningful when aging adults are younger, but also when they are very old.

One's present-day experience with nature does not have to be exactly the same as past experiences. Marlette's husband Brian had a beautiful grandmother named Kathleen. Always a lover of nature, in Kathleen's very old age it was necessary for her to go into a care facility. She stated that she needed only one thing: a bed beside a window, with a tree outside that window. She got this, and she enjoyed the changing of seasons, the birds that came to rest in that tree, and the leaves rustling in the wind; in this way and others, she nourished her soul. Her present-day experience of nature evoked past memories and feelings, and her soul was satisfied.

QUESTIONS TO PONDER:
- What aspects of your life do you find mundane?
- What meaning do you find in the ordinary?

- What can you do to wrest meaning from your mundane?

Tips for Consideration:
- At the beginning of the day, purpose within yourself that you will look for meaning throughout your daily work, tasks, and activities.
- When you discover something you find meaningful, write down what was meaningful and why it was meaningful to you.
- Also write down how the recognition of something meaningful impacted your day.

chapter four

FINDING MEANING
IN UNEXPECTED PLACES

Even though I walk through the valley of the shadow of death, I fear no evil, for You are with me; Your rod and Your staff, they comfort me.
                                                    —Psalm 23:4 (NASB)

If there is meaning in life at all, then there must be meaning in suffering.
                                                    —Viktor Frankl
                            Holocaust survivor and Austrian psychiatrist
                                                    (Goodreads, 2016c)

Throughout this book, we assert that meaning is extremely important, particularly to aging adults. We also note that meaning can be found in faith communities or spiritual beliefs. That being said, we also contend that older adults sometimes hold fast to their spiritual beliefs and yet feel profoundly empty. They may wonder where they can find meaning if they cannot find it where they once did. What once worked, for one reason or another, no longer does. In this chapter, however, we suggest that while meaning can be found in expected places, it is sometimes wrapped up in unwelcome circumstances. And although meaning may be difficult to find or laborious to sustain, at times we may be so jarred by life's essence that we become open to meaning in the different facets of our lives; that which once was meaningful, but then seemed to lose meaning, is again infused with meaning through the unexpected experience.

HARD WORK

Hard work, is, well, hard! It is often exhausting and challenging and may stretch us physically and mentally as we try to persevere. Some may believe that meaning does not come from hard work because of their belief that meaning should somehow emanate easily from life, circumstances, or spiritual beliefs. In this book, we are attempting to debunk this belief, or at least expose it as a partial myth.

It is true that many of us can remember a time sitting in a place of worship, attending a wedding, or listening to a moving piece of music when we felt a sense of meaning and connection to something much greater than ourselves. We truly did little work to feel this sense of meaning. However, that moment of *meaning clarity* was brief; it was gone almost as quickly as it came. True, an emotional response to that sense of meaning might have lasted for a few days, but it quickly vanished with the cares of everyday life. We may have found ourselves trying to recreate this sense of meaning through similar circumstances, but we were not able to do so. One man said, in describing his entrance into a sacred space, "I could just feel the Presence!" While this experience was arresting and nourishing to his soul, and while he could draw upon it as a memory from time to time, it has not been enough to sustain his soul in the day-to-day grind of life.

Wresting meaning out of everyday life involves work. It sounds so basic that one could question why it needs to be emphasized. However, by the time some folks reach their latter years, they have slowed to a state of inertia. Reading the news-paper and watching TV may be time-fillers, but they do not produce joy; getting out there and doing something meaningful can seem like

> Wresting meaning out of everyday life involves work.

moving a mountain. And for those individuals whose lives have been slowing for decades, they may no longer recognize what is meaningful for them. They may need to start the earthmover of their lives by getting in touch again with what brings them meaning.

For an example, we'll use the earthy metaphor quite literally. For some, it may mean working on the land, tending to stubborn animals, and shoveling manure. The work can be backbreaking (figuratively, of course) and obviously not suitable for the very old. However, it can be intensely meaningful. Working outside with the land (soil) gives one a sense of being part of nature and the universe. For some, this is profoundly significant in their lives and truly a part of how they conceptualize themselves. Hence, so many older adults work in their gardens or flowerbeds. When kneeling and bending become problematic, some work with flowerpots on windowsills, or plant a garden in a trug.[6]

Working with animals can also be extremely rewarding. For aging adults who volunteer at an animal shelter, tending to the animals and offering extra cuddles and attention to those in their care can move them beyond a self-focus. Through the act of nurturing animals in need of comfort, they experience the joy of giving; the reward is not monetary, and when it comes it is in the form of a grateful, responsive animal. But it is amazingly powerful!

DISAPPOINTMENTS

It is sometimes assumed that younger individuals have a greater challenge coping with disappointments than other age groups, but we say that older adults can experience painful disappointments that are even harder to confront and work through. For instance, some individuals realize in their fifties or sixties that dreams they held dear, dreams they never acted upon but always planned to, will never come to fruition. Sometimes these unrealized dreams cannot be attained; for instance, a woman in her late fifties cannot have a child by natural means. This can be devastating. Aging individuals can start to question if their lives have had meaning in terms of what they wanted to do, their impact upon others, their community, or the world.

---

6 In this sense, we are referring to an elevated trough in which one can grow flowers or vegetables. For those in apartments, or for those who cannot bend deeply, they can still get the sense of their hands in the soil, and receive products for their efforts.

Disappointments may be viewed as antithetical to meaning. However, coming face to face with disappointments may actually lead to new and different kinds of meaning. Disappointments cause people to call into question their beliefs. If what they hoped for did not come to pass, aging individuals need to consider, what now? "What do I believe and how do I make sense of these beliefs in relation to my life experiences?"

If I believed that I could avoid chronic illness through healthy behaviors, and now I have significant pain related to osteoarthritis and Type 2 diabetes, how do I adapt my beliefs without feeling despair? While this example may seem trite, many have molded their lives (not entirely unreasonably) around beliefs that if they exercised, ate right, took vitamins, and followed other rules, they would remain healthy in their later years. The disappointment of this not occurring has led to embarrassment (as they counseled their friends on how to take care of themselves) and created an unsettling sense of loss of control. At this point, the question becomes, "How do I go forward now and make the most of my last years?" Or, more simply for some, "What will I do now that I cannot play golf?" If the illness is progressive, there may be a struggle with chronic sorrow: "I've lost my ability to play golf because of osteoarthritis. Could I lose my sight as well, because of the diabetes? Then I won't even be able to watch golf on TV..."

It does not mean that they will not grieve the disappointments; the pain can remain for some time. However, aging adults can be challenged to assess who they are as individuals, what values and beliefs they hold dear, and how they can practically act on those values to make a difference. They can consider how old passions that were set aside due to other interests or demands can be rein-corporated into the present.

For instance, an older adult who is now unable to assist in volunteering for humanitarian efforts overseas may reestablish his love of books and children by volunteering to read to kids at the local library. This act stitches the past into the present in a way that represents his values, beliefs, and personhood, enhancing the beauty of his tapestry.[7]

DEALINGS WITH DIFFICULT PEOPLE

For some of us, dealing with difficult people is one of life's largest challenges. These individuals may be good people, but something about them—their ideas or how they act toward us—is off-putting. How can these individuals nudge us towards finding or sustaining meaning in life? In part, difficult people, for whatever reason, cause us to reflect on what it is that grates on us. If their opinions or beliefs are offensive, we may reflect upon why we believe or react as we do. If it is their manner of expression that is distasteful, we consider what is specifically bothersome and how our comportment differs. We may even consider how what we say or do impacts others, and if others may find us offensive.

If we are inclined to contemplation in relation to ourselves and others, we may even consider how our ideas and beliefs may be processed and understood in light of

---

7 See Chapter Five for a discussion of how family members or friends can help older adults, including conducting a mini life review of meaning with their loved ones.

the beliefs of others. How is it that others may be good people but believe so differently than ourselves? The process of reflection can be meaningful. We not only consider our beliefs in relation to others, but we may look for areas of commonality. Through this reflection upon our own lives, brought about by the impact of difficult people, we may refine some of our own thoughts and behaviors. We may experience empathy for these individuals and a deeper sense of value in our beliefs and choices. As Socrates is credited to have said, "The unexamined life is not worth living" (BrainyQuotes, 2016e). The impact of difficult others may propel us into an examined life, and hence enhance our life's meaning.

HEALTH CHALLENGES

In a previous book (Lane & Reed, 2015), we discussed how health challenges for older adults are transitions which can result in existential issues, or issues related to meaning and purpose. Older adults can wonder what the purpose of life is when they cannot do what they once could. This is especially important because we largely define ourselves in society by what we do (profession) rather than who we are (a grandmother of five, for example). Further, in the western world, we stubbornly cling to the notion of independence rather than interdependence. Thus, when older adults need assistance with activities of everyday life, they may feel they are too much of a burden to their family, friends, and community.

We understand how older adults may experience this sense of hopelessness and of being burdensome to family.

However, we believe that health challenges can be a vehicle for finding meaning, albeit in an unexpected way.

Dr. Jennifer Bute is a retired family physician who has early-stage dementia. She recently wrote an article about strategies for living with dementia and concludes that it is a gift and an opportunity for the faith community to demonstrate God's love (2016). Certainly, we doubt that she would have chosen to experience dementia, but God's love is evident to her through her illness (giving meaning), and in her account she suggested how those in the faith community can respond helpfully. We offer that Bute may find meaning in her illness as she identifies how God continues to be with her and how she can help others understand dementia. We also propose that her illness provides meaning to those who care for her or minister to her. They are confronted with a situation they would not choose and then they consider (even wrestle with) how their theology of God's love would work for them if they were in the same situation. They also find comfort in fulfilling the Golden Rule—doing unto Dr. Bute as they would have had her do unto them.

Similarly, MacKinlay (2016) presented her journey with a friend who is experiencing dementia. As a nurse and Anglican priest, she discussed how theology can work in relation to helping someone with dementia. She outlined the importance of listening to the stories of those with dementia, hearing their comments, which can be imbued with wisdom, and helping them to connect with God even when their cognition has significantly deteriorated. She also illustrated the importance of connecting with her significantly demented mother, whether or not her mother realizes that she is her daughter. MacKinlay (2016) asserted that those with dementia experience meaning and can be insightful; she also contended that those who help them experience meaning through a stretching of their own faith paradigms (God can be real to individuals even in a decline of cognition).

Marlette provided spiritual care for a man who had both dementia and schizophrenia. He'd often say to her, as nurses were sharing a joke outside of his room, "They're laughing at me, aren't they?" At other times, he'd point out to her the people who were coming through the walls of his room. Jim and Marlette had developed a trusting relationship over a period of time, and while these symptoms were not always present, they were not uncommon. To his expressed fears about staff laughing at him, Marlette would respond, "They are enjoying each other's company outside your room, but they aren't laughing at you, Jim." Regarding the individuals coming through the walls, Jim would see her face and say, "Oh, I guess they're not really there." "No, Jim, they're not." There was much respect and love between this elderly gentleman and Marlette; he honored her with his confidences. She was never so honored as when he'd respond, "I need to trust more." And when they would pray together at the end of his visit (he always wanted to), he would pray, "God, help me to trust You more!" Marlette was always humbled in hearing Jim pray; the challenges of his mind were profound, and rather than rejecting his faith he continued to reach out. If he could trust in his circumstances, could she not reach out more in trusting God? In this relationship, she found her own faith stretched, and her respect for Jim deepened.

Annette M. Lane and Marlette B. Reed

CHANGES IN LIVING ENVIRONMENT

We hesitate to address finding meaning in changes in living environment, as we ourselves have never experienced having to move to an environment that was avoided or feared. For older adults, this dreaded environment may involve a move to a nursing home. Such a move can represent great loss for aging adults, and indeed, a significant move closer towards death.

Interestingly, a body of research is emerging that examines how older adults find meaning in their moves to other living locations, such as nursing homes. Recent work by Haugan (2014a) has confirmed the importance of meaning in coping with life in institutional facilities. Meaning in life is connected to one's emotional well-being and functional ability (Haugan, 2014b) in nursing homes, not just to when older adults live independently in the community. Simply put, older adults who are able to glean meaning in this change of environment may experience better physical, mental, and functional health.

In an interesting study, Dwyer and colleagues (2008) interviewed three women living in nursing homes in Sweden. These women addressed how they found meaning despite challenges such as blindness and being wheelchair-bound; one woman was confined to her bed. For these women, meaning came from interactions, conversations, and connections with others. Also, they experienced meaning through their inner dialogue—in essence, their self-talk. One woman looked at family pictures in her room and thought about her roles as mother and grandmother and reflected with great enjoyment on these responsibilities. Another aging woman who had never had children reflected upon her resilience and that she had always been a fighter. This woman continued to be greatly interested in societal issues such as class differences and women's rights and wanted to speak with others about these matters. Both women were self-soothing; they were nourishing their souls!

Another very important point coming from the study of Dwyer and her colleagues (2008) involved how these women wanted to be seen. One woman spoke about wanting staff in the nursing home to see her as she conceptualized herself, not necessarily as they saw her. This woman was expressing the importance of her individuality and the meaning she derived from personhood. Our personhood can therefore bring us meaning; the challenge, however, can be to express that personhood (soul) in a way that is congruent with how we perceive ourselves, rather than how others see us.

For instance, a person with a chronic illness may view himself as a vital, healthy, and contributing member of society. He feels this way even though his legs no longer do the job for him and he is in a wheelchair. This gentleman may experience great frustration in trying to move

> Our personhood can therefore bring us meaning; the challenge, however, can be to express that personhood (soul) in a way that is congruent with how we perceive ourselves, rather than how others see us.

others away from pity towards respect for who he is as a man. But in doing this, he may both limit the chronic sorrow he experiences (losses heaped upon each other) and instruct others in how to view him and perhaps even other individuals with mobility challenges. For example, this fellow may not be able to get out of his wheelchair, but he can still maneuver it with his arms. Rather than submitting to being pushed in his chair, he may say to a well-meaning woman who wants to push him, "Thanks, but I like to do this myself. Working my arms increases my upper body strength." So he gets the exercise, defines the limits of his disability for himself and the other person, and demonstrates his moxie, his chutzpah, as a man who still can do many things.

DYING AND DEATH

Discussing dying and death is considered macabre in our society. Addressing the fact that our lives are finite and that each of us is moving towards death appears strange and antithetical to social discourse (how we talk about our daily lives). However, it is important to consider that dying and death is truly a part of life, and that profound meaning can be experienced in dying and death. In Marlette's time as a palliative care chaplain, she had the privilege of working with hundreds of dying older adults and their family members. Her work absolutely convinced her of the meaning that can be wrested through dying and death.

A REFOCUS ON THAT WHICH IS REALLY IMPORTANT
For most of us, our lives are dictated by activities that are necessary or enjoyable for everyday life but not necessarily connected with meaning, spirituality, or God. We may honestly try to incorporate meaning, faith, and spirituality in our lives, but we often slip into the routine without recognizing meaning in the mundane (Chapter Three).

A crisis like finding out we are ill or dying, or that a loved one is dying, confronts us with a different reality. The new reality (the "anticipated endings" addressed by Fredrickson and Carstensen, 1998) impacts our life vision in a couple of ways. First, the things that seemed so important—a disagreement with a neighbor, keeping up with our friends in terms of trips or cars—now seem misguided and inconsequential. We may wonder how we could have been so shortsighted; we have miswanted (Gilbert & Wilson, 2000). Secondly, confronting our own mortality, or that of loved ones, challenges us to consider our life paradigm, including what we find meaningful in life. The "meaning" that came from buying a new car now seems shallow and insufficient for facing into our reality. Suddenly, we are scrambling to get in touch with our belief system, which may have lost its muscle over the years, or find some new meaning in our current situation. If not, we may wonder if our lives have been in vain and may pass away in great existential angst.

While it is generally understood that people in difficult circumstances find comfort in faith and spirituality (hence the term "foxhole religion"), studies also show that religion and/or spirituality bring meaning to those who grieve the loss of a spouse. Initially, grieving people can feel spiritually lost; they are no longer the spouse of their partner, so who are they?

"Who am I?" is a profoundly spiritual question! Spiritual practices—religious rituals or going to a gravesite, for example—enhance grieving; spiritual beliefs help those who grieve realize that though the relationship is different, it still carries on, whether the loved one is "in heaven" or "always with them". Spirituality aids in helping those who have lost one they love to come to a sense of new identity (Damianakis & Marziali, 2012). As religion and spirituality are all about meaning, the lenses through which we process such an enormous loss, as well as the supports needed to carry those who are grieving (such as spiritual and religious practices), can greatly aid the surviving spouse.

Reconnection with Family and Friends

Dying and death reconnect us with family and friends we might rarely see. We may have lost touch because of geographical distance, dissimilar interests, work constraints, or misunderstandings. Standing at the bedside or graveside of a shared loved one forces us to converse and immediately thrusts us into intimate situations where tears may be shed, apologies offered, and reconnections occur. Not only is this extremely comforting in our grief following the passing of a loved one, it also reminds us that there is more to life than activities for the sake of activities; we remember the worth and meaning in connecting with and standing together with others. We may also take comfort that some good has come out of dreadful circumstances.

Deepening Relationships with Family and Friends

In day-to-day living, our relationships can become perfunctory. Yes, we appreciate those in our lives, but sometimes we may relate to them in superficial ways. When a crisis occurs due to the hospitalization of a spouse, a friend might drop what she was doing, meet you at the hospital, and spend hours with you. Not only does this friend talk gently to your spouse, hold his hand, and calm him when he becomes restless, but she spends time pacing the hospital floors with you. You always valued this friendship, but the level of appreciation deepens tremendously. You now cherish this person, as she has been willing to support you in your darkest time and is not afraid of how to be with you, particularly in the silences where nothing is said. In the difficult circumstances, you see the depth of her personhood, the graciousness of heart, and her wonderful commitment towards you. While you obviously did not wish for this very bleak time, the strength of her personhood and friendship comforts you when later your spouse passes. You also know that this is a friend who will listen to your grief in the coming months; she has become your foxhole buddy.

THE INVITATION TO FIND MEANING IN THE MUNDANE
When we face our own death or that of a loved one, mundane activities may become more meaningful. Why? There are several reasons. First, we may be grateful that we can still do some aspects of self-care. Preparing soup from a can may seem like a gift we no longer take for granted. Second, the mundane becomes the context through which others—such as friends, family, and colleagues—connect to us by assisting us in a meaningful way. When they validate us through their assistance and verbal and physical expressions of kindness and care, we are strengthened and find meaning in what was once considered ordinary; a meal dropped by the house is not just food in a dish, it is an expression of love. Third, when we can only lie on a couch or in a hospital bed, we may take great joy in that which is so basic.

We spoke earlier of a person's inner boundaries expanding as their outer boundaries shrink. For a person in a hospice bed, a few sips of an icy cold milkshake can be exhilarating! The tender hand of a compassionate nurse is soul-nourishing, the laughs shared with a gracious volunteer so meaningful that these chuckles can bring the dying individual to tears. Rather than gulping life in macro proportions, it is savored in micro quantities.

WHOLENESS WHERE THE PIECES HAVE BEEN BROKEN

No matter how carefully we have tried to live purposefully and meaningfully, inevitably, most of us have regrets. We may regret cherished relationships that have turned sour or goals we have not reached and now realize we will never reach. Finding a sense of completeness in these situations is important in the dying process, and indeed, can bring great meaning to this process.

With time running out, dying people often desire to put their affairs in order. Perhaps easiest are the legal and financial things; wills are written and outstanding bills are paid, for example. (It must be stated, however, that more than one widow has discovered the family finances in a mess!) The work often lays in one's sense of completion within self, relationships, and God.

Within the self, one often has to come to grips with regrets in life: "If I could do it all over again, I'd do this, not that." Sometimes, the failing older adult feels that the best way of rectifying this is the extraction of a promise from an adult child to do or not do something. This is generally not effective. The "if onlys" and "should have, could have, would haves" are often best talked out with someone in the older adult's life, someone who can bring some perspective. The mini life review can be a helpful exercise, as discussed in Chapter Five.

Where the regrets have more to do with hurts caused or relationships severed, an exercise in forgiveness can be helpful. If one is a person of faith, this can be facilitated through a religious ritual. If there is no faith through which to process the need to receive forgiveness (from self, others, or the Other), the act of confession to a trusted person, chaplain, or counselor, and realistic discussion about what can be done about this area of brokenness, can help to bring some sense of integrity, of wholeness. The seeking of forgiveness becomes the gold or silver that beautifully melds together broken pieces.

And people often (re)turn to the faith of their childhood. It would seem that whatever was hardwired onto the computer of the soul is (re)accessed as death approaches. The need to prepare oneself for the next life is often at the root of this. As well, aging individuals often approach the day-to-day in a spiritual way, as addressed already, in order to squeeze out meaning, so that they can both wrest and rest. Faith and spirituality foster hope and "hope fuels the energy to face suffering and to make meaning through times of great pain" (Groot-Alberts, 2012, p, 161). Chapter Six will address the soul work of end-of-life in more depth.

FINDING MEANING IN GRATITUDE

In this chapter, we have focused largely upon negative life situations: circumstances that most of us dread. As such, talking about finding meaning in gratitude, which usually is associated with positive events, seems incongruous. However, gratitude does fit in a chapter that addresses meaning in difficult circumstances. When we find reasons to be grateful, even in unwanted conditions or happenings, we lessen the impact of trauma upon ourselves. We open our eyes to what good may come out of a bad situation, such as new relationships or opportunities, and we maintain enough perspective to cope. This is not to say that we welcome the circumstances, but rather we acknowledge that in painful situations, we can find a few things for which to be grateful.

Gratitude is a virtue extolled in many world religions. As has often been acknowledged, the Apostle Paul wrote, *"No matter what happens, always be thankful, for this is God's will for you who belong to Christ Jesus"* (1 Thessalonians 5:18, TLB); he wrote this when his life circumstances were perpetually dire. His ministry was beset with difficulties, such as stoning, shipwrecks, and imprisonment.

In the last fifteen years, gratitude has become a focus of psychology; there are books, websites, and institutes dedicated to this topic. American philosopher and journalist A.J. Jacobs, who is an agnostic, spoke in his TED-Talk entitled "My year of living biblically" (2008) about how giving thanks changed him profoundly:

I was praying... these prayers of thanksgiving.... I was saying thanks all the time, every day, and I started to change my perspective. And I started to realize the hundreds of little things that go right every day... as opposed to focusing on the three or four that went wrong.

This biblical encouragement towards gratitude may seem preposterous when life is really difficult, yet gratitude facilitates perspective, which aids in finding meaning and thereby enhances resilience.

QUESTIONS TO PONDER:

- Think about the disappointments in your life. How have they impacted how you view yourself?
- How have disappointments influenced a sense of meaning in your life and your understanding and experience of God?
- How can you find meaning in the unexpected places in your life?

TIPS FOR CONSIDERATION:

- After considering the above questions, write down your findings. In particular, document what meaning you experienced in unexpected circumstances. How has the meaning gained from these circumstances (e.g., personality development, empathy, resilience, new talents) impacted your life in the years following?
- If you have a trusted other with whom you can speak about difficult past experiences, share your discoveries with them. What does this individual say about the meaning or good that may have come out of your past difficulties and how that has continued to help you in your life?

chapter five

HELPING OLDER ADULTS FIND MEANING

Two can accomplish more than twice as much as one, for the results can be much better. If one falls, the other pulls him up; but if a man falls when he is alone, he's in trouble.

—Ecclesiastes 4:9–10 (TLB)

Let no one ever come to you without leaving better and happier.

Never worry about numbers. Help one person at a time, and always start with the person nearest you.

—Mother Teresa
founder of the Missionaries of Charity
(Quotegarden.com, 2016b)

In our younger adult years, finding and sustaining meaning is in many ways our own responsibility. Generally speaking, we have the health and ability to decide our values, our goals, and how we derive meaning. As we enter our later years, our ability to sustain meaning in day-to-day living may slowly or suddenly decline due to physical or mental challenges. As such, we may need to look to family members, relatives, or friends to help us in our quest to maintain meaning in our lives. This does not mean we become totally passive; we too must engage in our quest to find and sustain the essence of life. The importance of meaning cannot be overstated due to its positive impact upon mental and physical health, as well as life satisfaction.

A television commercial may illustrate the importance of helping aging adults find and sustain meaning. A 2015 car commercial portrayed a farmer who was going to herd his sheep. As he approached his vehicle to drive to the field, he looked back and saw his border collie hobbling (with a cast on one front paw) and looking expectantly at his master. The dog wanted to fulfill his usual duties of herding sheep! In the farmer's eyes, there was momentary hesitation. It appeared like he was unsure if he wanted to take his dog. After a brief moment, the farmer made a decision and scooped up his collie into his arms, placing him in the back seat. He drove to the field and guided the sheep with his car while the dog stuck his head out of the window and barked furiously and triumphantly at the sheep. The look of satisfaction and pride in the dog's eyes was very moving.

In watching this commercial, we thought about aging adults. They need to be involved in important matters in their latter years; this does not change from when they were younger, yet sometimes they need assistance to make meaningful work happen. This is where family members, relatives, and friends can make a significant difference. So what can family and friends do to assist their aging loved ones? We offer some suggestions below.

ACKNOWLEDGE THEIR
WORTH AS HUMAN BEINGS

At all stages of life, human beings need to feel loved and valued. Felt love enables us to experience some security in this world and promotes a sense of being valued. The need to feel loved and valued does not diminish with age; for some individuals, this need grows stronger as other sources of validation, such as their profession or ability to perform physical feats are no longer available to them. It is therefore very important that as family members, or friends of older adults, you endorse their worth. Tell them that you love and appreciate them, not just for what they did in the past, but also for what they do and who they are in the present. This involves being specific about what you see in them as individuals, such as personality traits, and what you have learned, and continue to learn, from them. Don't assume that they know you love them or that their memories of the past are enough to sustain them in the present.

LOOK FOR THEIR BEAUTY

At the beginning of this book, we spoke of North American society's emphasis on youth and its attractiveness. As we live in this type of culture, we may need to train ourselves to widen our understanding. Consider the words of Elisabeth Kubler-Ross:

> *The most beautiful people... are those who have known defeat... suffering... struggle... loss, and have found their way out of the depths. These persons have an appreciation, a sensitivity, and an*

understanding of life that fills them with com-passion, gentleness, and a deep loving concern.
(Goodreads, 2016d)

The fact that your elderly parent has lived a long time guarantees that they will have known suffering. In what ways have they overcome? How did they overcome? How do they demonstrate compassion towards others? By adjusting your lenses for beauty, you will likely see some pretty amazing qualities in them. An individual who has compassion, gentleness, and love in their soul, having overcome much, is beautiful! Understanding what your elderly loved one has gone through may give you a heightened appreciation for who they are, and help you to value them that much more.

Does one only value the parent who has "found their way out of the depths" and become beautiful? What about the elderly parent whose struggles did not lead to beauty of character? Valuing that parent is understandably more difficult. And in this case, some wise adult children have chosen to see the struggles their parents came through, understanding that they are broken, and value them for who they are in God's sight—priceless.

HOLDING SPACE

This wonderful concept is often used in palliative care, but it can be utilized in many of life's challenges. To hold space for someone means to journey with them in an accepting, non-judgmental way; we do not try to "fix" them, or the situation, but with our presence, we provide the space for them to grieve, try new things, and be vulnerable. It means not insisting upon the outcome of our company (Plett, 2016).

At one time, parents held space for their children. When a child fell and hurt herself, her parents were a safe place for her to run to; they provided care and did not shame her for her tears. In that held space, the young girl was able to draw strength and carry on with the knowledge that she was loved. That same girl may later in life need to hold space for her elderly parents. If one of them falls and breaks a bone, she may need to come over and help that parent with bathing, meal preparation, and listening to the story of the fall, sometimes repeatedly. Likely behind that story is some shame ("How could I have been so stupid to trip on that step?") and fear ("What if your father hadn't been home to call 911?"). In her vulnerability, the one who once mothered—holding space—now is on the receiving end of that type of care. Adult children will marvel at how, over the course of their lives, the roles have changed.

> To hold space for someone means to journey with them in an accepting, non-judgmental way; we do not try to "fix" them, or the situation, but with our presence, we provide the space for them to grieve, try new things, and be vulnerable.

CONNECT WITH THEM

While the concepts of valuing our elders and holding space have significant spiritual and emotional components, connecting with them incorporates the valuable aspects of time, as well as frequency. It is easier to connect with older adults who live near to you. And yet as aging relatives need more instrumental help (with buying groceries, doing yardwork, or paying bills, as examples), the focus of the visits often becomes the tasks at hand. While this is under-standable, it should not be the only reason to see your loved one. If your visits are centered on tasks, try to incorporate a cup of coffee at the mall or in your loved one's kitchen. As difficult as it can be, try to remain relaxed while visiting. It is so easy—we know from personal experience—to be thinking about all the other tasks and work that needs to be done. All of us who have assisted older loved ones have felt the pangs of guilt from having rushed those we love, perhaps giving the message that we are too busy.

Even if you are geographically separated from this older family member, advances in technology allow you to not only talk with an aging loved one, but also to see him or her. While aging adults may not have grown up with computers and related technology, some are incred-ibly adept. Annette has a colleague who skypes with her ninety-six-year-old mother! We think this is wonderful. Not only can this colleague and her mother talk with each other, they can even see each other. Technology does not replace face-to-face contact, which allows for touch and the sense of being in the other's presence, but certainly it keeps a sense of connection.

WHERE POSSIBLE, HELP THEM CONNECT WITH OTHERS

As individuals age, their abilities to connect with others may be compromised through physical changes such as decreased vision or hearing. Helping an older adult may be as simple as driving the individual to an appointment for a hearing aid or taking that person to an eye examination. Better hearing or vision may result in this aging person feeling more connected to the world and hence re-energized and wanting to reengage.

Some aging adults may be unable to drive or feel uncomfortable driving long distances. Thus, enabling older adults to connect with others may involve getting them set up with a taxi service for older persons (with reduced rates) or driving them to friends or events. One dear older lady lost a cherished cousin in a distant town; she wanted badly to attend the funeral but could not drive long distances. Her son volunteered to take her. This trip would involve extended time in the car with her beloved son, honoring her deceased cousin, and connecting with other family members at the funeral whom she had not seen in years. While the passing of her cousin brought sadness, the funeral and the activities surrounding it provided her with connection, meaning, and engagement.

Helping aging adults connect with others becomes more significant as they become very old. As their contemporaries pass away, reconnecting with people they have known in the past, as well as making new friends, is crucial in sustaining a sense of meaning (Jonsen et al., 2015).

DISCUSSION ON MEANING IN LIFE

If you suspect that an older adult you know is feeling bored or aimless, talk to this person about it. Does your parent, spouse, or friend recognize that he is bored? Although we sometimes think that it should be obvious when a person is feeling bored and unstimulated by life, this is not always the case. In one seminar we conducted, a thoughtful older man spoke with us afterwards and stated "Now I know I am bored!" He had not recognized his experience as one of boredom but had, perhaps, framed this as aging or fatigue.

If you suspect an aging loved one is feeling a sense of meaningless or detachment from living, engage him or her in a mini life review of what has given meaning throughout life. You can ask your loved one about what activities gave her meaning in the past. Was it the connection to other like-minded individuals? Did he find it meaningful to be connected to an organization that was doing work he valued, such as feeding the poor, providing water wells for villages in Africa, or increasing literacy in developing countries? How can he or she reconnect with former sources of meaning? While you may remember that your dad belonged to a service club, you may not know what it was about that involvement that brought him meaning. This information helps you to know your father better; it also aids you in helping him find meaning in the present.

If the sources of meaning have remained the same, but the aging adult is less able to engage in these activities because of changes in health or transportation issues, creatively think of other ways that the individual can remain engaged with these organizations/groups. Or think about similar kinds of organizations or groups the aging adult can connect with that are perhaps closer to home. In our other book (Lane & Reed, 2015), we spoke at length about studies examining the benefits of volunteering and a wide range of volunteer activities, such as volunteering online, being a phone support for and mentor of aging adults (as an older individual), physically going to agencies and volunteering, and being part of an activist group to lobby the government for changes to help those with AIDS in Africa. This in no way diminishes the importance of volunteering within churches, but for some older adults, working within communities that share the same faith is not enough.

If you are conversing with an older loved one and this person cannot identify what would give them meaning now, be prepared to speak to his or her talents, personality strengths, life focus, and others parts of personhood. You might recognize that your older family member is a mentor, not just to her grandchildren or nieces and nephews, but also to a couple of children in the neighborhood. It is useful for you to name the contribution for what it is: a contribution to the family, as well as to society. Often, aging individuals who provide excellent mentorship for younger generations do not recognize the worth of and skills involved in their work.

For instance, when attending university, Marlette's son Jon would occasionally drop by his aunt Annette's office in the nursing faculty. Working on his undergraduate degree, Jon would sometimes speak about what he was going to do with his life. Though six-foot-four and burly (a weightlifter), he sought out his older and physically much smaller aunt for her advice and experience, because she was one step removed from his parents, who were highly invested in his career choices. Was it meaningful advice? Annette certainly hopes so, and Marlette states it was very helpful! Overall, however, the point of this example is that Jon's aunt understands her nephew, his strengths and talents, as well as how he is wired emotionally. Annette could speak to this and offer advice based upon her knowledge of Jon; she could also be a safe and less invested person to consult in terms of the outcome! Interestingly, the experience was meaningful for Annette because the action of her nephew seeking her out and asking advice indicated that her nephew respects and trusts her. This is high praise indeed!

HELP OLDER ADULTS
FULFILL THEIR COMMITMENTS

Increasingly, not-for-profit agencies and businesses want their volunteers to commit to a particular amount of volunteer time. This is understandable, as these agencies often train their volunteers and provide perks or benefits for their work. A stable cadre of volunteers is part of the successful running of not-for-profit agencies. In order to facilitate the ability of older adults to honor their commitment to volunteer work, family members or friends may need to help out with rides (e.g., driving when the taxi cannot come), encouragement, or other means of support. Recognize that this work is more than "just volunteer work." The work may be the means through which your older loved one grabs hold of meaning and sustains it. It also is the means through which aging adults can connect with others, particularly others who appreciate what they are doing. And from a broader perspective, your aging adult continues to make an important difference in the world.

In helping your aging loved ones find and sustain meaning, there may be points in their lives when activities have to be scaled back due to health or other circumstances. In these situations, you may need to help them find meaning in other ways. We have found that when our aging loved ones were no longer able to volunteer or engage deeply in life due to cognitive impairment, the most we could do was take them out for coffee or a meal. In these situations, we tried to tell a funny story to evoke a smile or laughter. Through our presence, tone of voice, words, and touch, we tried to convey that we loved them, that they were important to us, and that we were glad they were in our lives.

So What Does This All Mean for Me?

As you work with your older parent, family member, or friend, issues might arise within yourself. You may understandably ask, "So what does this mean for me?" We suggest that your work in helping older loved ones can mean a significant amount to you now and in the future.

Meaning in Helping Older Adults Now

Witness their strengths and struggles. There is a tremendous privilege in bearing witness to the struggles and triumphs of our loved ones, including those who are aging. Sometimes the most courageous moments in individuals' lives come in quiet, unobserved, day-to-day living. When we take the arm of an aging relative, who is unsteady on her feet, to walk into the hospital for some type of treatment, and she makes a witty joke as well as thanks us for our help, we see both her struggle and triumph. Though poor of health, her spirit is courageous; witty and gracious, she reveals the largesse of her heart. Even in her slow, unsteady gait, she carries herself with an air of dignity. To observe that quiet courage is a privilege indeed!

Not only is it an honor to witness our aging loved ones press on despite physical and sometimes cognitive challenges, it teaches us how to persevere through difficult times, including when we age. In this day and age, with our emphasis on ease, we can become seduced into believing that life should be relatively trouble-free and painless. Yet life is not smooth and comfortable. When aging adults respond to hardships and pain with a strong desire to live and eke out as much joy and meaning in life as they can, they serve as powerful teachers to younger generations. What they teach us—that there is joy and meaning in life not just in spite of the pain, but sometimes because of the pain—is incredibly profound and needed in our society.

In one of our recent seminars, we saw a woman our parents knew and greatly appreciated many years ago. In fact, even though we had lost touch, this dear woman came to our mother's funeral. When Marlette saw her, the two hugged. At one point in their conversation, this dear very elderly woman commented that she did not know why she was still here, as many of her contemporaries had passed. And yet this woman continues to do enormous good in her church and in the world around her. She is truly beautiful, inside and outside. Her focus on honoring God and others has preserved her dignity and grace. Using Elisabeth Kubler-Ross' statement quoted earlier in this chapter, her overcoming has produced in her great beauty!

> What they teach us - that there is joy and meaning in life not just in spite of the pain, but sometimes because of the pain - is incredibly profound and needed in our society.

In witnessing your older adult's strengths and struggles through helping him, you may also have the opportunity to hear stories about situations that impacted him when he was young. Your aging parent or relative may talk about the war and his experiences, or a lengthy period of time spent in hospital during childhood, or the extreme poverty he and his siblings endured. You may then ask questions about his childhood that allows him to reminisce and also answers questions you may have of your heritage.

We both wish we had asked our parents more questions about our heritage and relatives. We listened with interest in their stories, but when we were young, they were just nice stories. They were not particularly significant to us. When our parents had both passed, we tried to access more information about relatives and illnesses in our family but did not find answers. We now wish we had asked more questions earlier, yet when we were in our thirties we had too many interests, commitments, and responsibilities to foster interest in the past. We also were looking to the future rather than reflecting upon the past.

Fulfill some of your needs for meaning, including giving back to those who gave so much to you. Most of us have a need for meaning throughout our lives. When we support our aging loved ones in finding and sustaining meaning, we capture some of life's essence ourselves. This is not to say that supporting aged loved ones over a lengthy period is easy; in fact, it can be exhausting, particularly when we are juggling our own work, family, and friends. However, it can be deeply meaningful to care for those who cared for us as we grew up. In a way, it gives us a sense of something larger than ourselves; as our parents cared for us when we were young, we care for them in their aging years, and hopefully our children or nieces and nephews will care for us. Thus our grandparents, parents, children, and nieces and nephews are part of a historical chain as well as the tapestry of our lives.

While being part of something much larger than ourselves may not be so important when we are young, as we age the historical elements of where our family came from, who we are in relation to our relatives, how we take up our ethnicities, and how our children or nieces/nephews carry on our family legacy become increasingly important and comforting. This sense of connection is truly spiritual.

Develops empathy and character. Supporting aging loved ones develops our character and sense of empathy. It forces us to think beyond ourselves and be concerned for others. While some are naturally focused on others, the tendency in today's world is to be "me-oriented." Having to think of others and sometimes put others first, despite our own inconvenience or cost, stretches us as people.

Developing empathy through helping aged family members helps us to develop an understanding of aging, so that we can help others who are assisting aging parents. It also produces in us a sensitivity to and understanding of the pain of seeing loved ones suffer, as well as the joy and pride of seeing them persevere. We can then cry with friends who cry about their parents and enter into their deep-seated pride over how one parent is providing exquisite care for the other; we can hold space. Our understanding of life—pain, joy, and meaning—expands, not just in regards to family members or friends but overall to situations and issues within society. It is as if we see life through new glasses—spiritual lenses. As we extend grace to others, we are better able to grant that same grace to ourselves. This can be so freeing!

MEANING IN THE FUTURE

It may teach you lessons about how to age productively. As you observe older family members aging, you are also learning how to age productively, or perhaps you may be observing less effective ways of aging. In truth, lessons can be learned from those we assist, whether they are experiencing positive aging or not. For instance, if you see an aging parent who is actively engaged in a faith community, is involved in a political party, fulfills contract work obligations, and helps neighbors with household/ yard tasks—showing that they are genuinely engaged and motivated by life—then you may learn the importance of having structure in your life upon retirement, as well as engagement in a variety of activities. You may also glean that being involved with others, not just in idle conversation but also in meaningful work, is what produces that genuine engagement. You might learn about the importance of becoming meaningfully involved in others' lives, even *before* you enter older age. If you get started in your quest for meaning prior to retirement and older age, you may nicely set yourself up for continuing meaning-making throughout your later years.

Conversely, if you see an aging relative who is embittered by years of disappointment and regret, you may resolve within yourself not to become that way. You might decide that you need to let go of some resentment towards others who have hurt you in the past; the jolt of seeing that relative so angry and disillusioned provides the impetus to change how you look at your life, including where you are now and what you want to be like in the future. Unintentionally, that relative has helped you enormously by his example, even if his illustration of aging has been negative.

One more thought about aging productively: by observing the differences between those who age well and those who struggle, you might take notice of how these individuals retired and began their first months and years in older adulthood. Did one of these individuals have meaning in his life prior to retirement, and what comprised that meaning? What did this individual do prior to retirement to build his capacity to engage in meaningful activity in his later years? What can you do now to start to prepare for your older years? Would it be helpful to talk with him about how he found and sustained meaning, particularly when faced with health challenges?

Help your grieving process when your loved aged is gone. Maya Angelou stated, "I've learned that regardless of your relationship with your parents, you'll miss them when they're gone from your life" (Goodreads, 2016e). Interesting quote, and some would certainly disagree! That being said, in this quote she pointed to an important aspect of life—that is, our lives and histories are ensconced in that of our parents. Our parents know their histories, to some degree, as well as ours. When they are gone, we can no longer ask them questions about when we were young, or about when they were young, or about their parents. Sadly, when we are young we may not care about such matters, but when we age, these details become more significant. We may have a greater need to understand what factors, seen and unseen, have shaped our lives.

And there is more. When we are young, or when we are adults caring for our aging parents, we may see their idiosyncrasies and faults. We may not understand what shaped them as parents (their upbringing) or the pressures they endured in trying to provide for their family. When they are gone and we are entering our fifties or sixties, we often garner a greater understanding of the pressures they experienced. Over time, we grasp what shaped their personalities and behaviors and feel much greater empathy, perhaps even admiration, for how they managed, despite their challenges. We might then feel some regret that we did not know or understand the impetus of their unhelpful behaviors (pressures such as war, mental health issues, or poverty in childhood). If we have provided care and support for them in their aging years, even if we did not understand their thoughts and actions, the memories of providing such care can bring us comfort. And those memories can bring us comfort when we grieve their loss.

Further, the times spent together helping aging parents can help us address issues of the past. For instance, we have worked with adults who came from homes where there was abuse, or where emotions such as love and compassion were not expressed. While they now understand what motivated a distant or abusive parent (mental illness, abandonment by their parents, etc.), they still feel a deep, gnawing emptiness and desire for approval. When providing assistance to a parent, the adult may receive spoken gratitude from that parent who previously was distant, or hear their parent voice apologies or the words "I love you." The expression of such sentiments is incredibly powerful! It does not erase the past, but it helps the adult child to leave the past in the past and move forward.

As this chapter comes to a close, we want to reiterate that sometimes, as noted in Chapter Two, adult children may not feel safe caring for an older parent. Their relationship with their parent may have been marred by abuse or neglect and adult children may truly feel traumatized, in the present, by helping their parent. In situations like these, we suggest that adult children seek the guidance of trusted others or professionals such as ministers or counselors.

Also, the adult children may choose not to be involved, or choose *how* to be involved. For instance, we have known situations where adult children managed the finances of the ailing parent, or washed clothes and brought cigarettes to the nursing home for the parent. These children were emotionally limited in how much time they could actually spend with their parent, but they wanted to honor the fact that this person was their parent biologically and respect that the parent was now a frail and failing older adult, not simply the person who had always frightened them. In this way, the adult children meet their own needs to honor their parent and also protect themselves. They also may experience great freedom as they recognize that in some ways they have moved on from their past.

QUESTIONS TO PONDER:
- How well do you know your parents in terms of what brings them meaning?
- What is/are one or both of your parents doing to foster meaning in aging?

- In what ways can you assist older adults in your life to find or sustain meaning-making and meaningful activities?

TIPS FOR CONSIDERATION:

- Reflect upon your answers to the questions above. If you determine that there are ways you could better assist parents or other older adults in your life, determine one or two ways you will help them find/sustain meaning.
- Talk with the older adult about your plans to help out.
- Follow through with this help, and in doing so reflect upon what you have learned through the processing of helping an aged individual find/sustain meaning.

chapter six

Your Life, Bringing the Pieces Together into a Work of Art

For I know the plans I have for you, says the Lord. They are plans for good and not for evil, to give you a future and a hope.
—Jeremiah 29:11 (TLB)

Whatever course you decide upon, there is always someone to tell you that you are wrong. There are always difficulties arising which tempt you to believe that your critics are right. To map out a course of action and follow it to an end requires courage.
—Ralph Waldo Emerson
American essayist and poet
(Quote Sea, 2016)

Throughout this book, we have addressed topics germane to making and sustaining meaning in our lives. We have offered reasons for why meaning-making is so important in older age and ways in which aging adults and their family members can make and sustain meaning. We recognize, however, that proposed ideas were scattered throughout the book, and therefore a reader may wonder,

"How do I get from point A (recognizing a lack of meaning) to point B (making or sustaining meaning)?" In this chapter, we discuss some ideas that have been developed throughout the book, particularly in Chapter Five. However, we address these ideas specifically for older adults rather than younger family members. As well, we consider these ideas in the context of tending to the past, living in the present, and looking toward the future. This is intentional living, along the same lines as the artist who restores the vase or the tapestry.

Remember the quote of Michael Drury (1988) with which we began this book:

> *A satisfactory life has to be* crafted... *one must see (old) age for what it is—a different mode and decide what one wants from it,* in it.... *An artist friend says if a man painted one masterpiece in his entire life, it was worth all his other effort.*
> (italics ours)

As long as a person lives, they have the opportunity to craft—to make, remake, make over, and make up.

Drury's quote speaks of the perspective of old age. One cannot, perhaps, recognize what constitutes a beautiful vase or tapestry in one's life until later in life. There may be an incredible achievement that one always feels proud of: military service for one's country, an award for an achievement, seeing one's children grow to become productive citizens and raise their own children to be productive, developing a bare piece of real estate into a beautiful property and home... the list is endless.

But people also have the opportunity to do significant work during their latter years, to bring meaning, to repair strains and ruptures in relationships, and to prepare for death. This too is invaluable. Gaining perspective on what is past and understanding in the present affords one the opportunity to work towards the future.

While dealing with specifics in putting one's life together—the masterpiece—in this chapter we focus strongly upon spiritual work. This focus will involve much Scripture and scriptural principles; as mentioned in the preface, it is our hope that as you have processed the language and research of the day on the subject of making meaning in older age, you will see the biblical teaching discussed in this chapter in a richer, more meaningful way than you may have previously.

IF POSSIBLE, START
EARLY IN MEANING-MAKING

While it is never too late to pursue meaning-making, we believe that it is helpful to incorporate it earlier rather than later. If you are an adult caring for aging parents, you might want to start now—even providing care for your parents is a means to finding meaning! As per the Drury quote, decide what it is you want from and in old age, and begin to apply yourself to that. Saving for the motorhome so that you and your partner can travel after retirement may be part of it, but this may be too big a goal to begin to work towards. Some people who think they may be headed in this direction start by renting a small motorhome from time to time, before they reach their senior years. In this way, one determines whether this dream of travelling is something both partners enjoy, how comfortable they feel in a small home twenty-four hours per day, and how expensive it is to live this way. Dreams require the necessary component of realism; taking measured and deliberate steps to realize them along the way is wise.

If you are a senior who is still working, the earlier you intentionally incorporate aspects of finding meaning in your life, the better. There are a couple of reasons for this. First, by starting early, you have time to try out different directions for making meaning (varied kinds of volunteer work, art work, a home business) and test what resonates with you. You might discover that one type of work appeals to you more than another. When you start earlier, your health is presumably better; time and good health allows for greater choice. Second, you may recognize how much richer your life feels earlier, and hence your sense of satisfaction may help you to sustain the behaviors involved in making meaning during retirement. The internal transition is already happening when one's actual retirement happens.

You may find it helpful to read Chapter Five again, particularly the questions (mini-review) that we suggested adult children raise with their parents. Spend some time reviewing what has given you meaning in the past. If you feel stumped in regards to what activities you might find meaningful, consult with a trusted friend. This friend may see qualities in you that you don't recognize, or, even if you do acknowledge these qualities, you may need help in understanding their worth!

In Your Basket of Meaning, Carry More than One Egg

As a concept, meaning encapsulates spirituality or faith, purposeful activities for the betterment of others, connection with others, and an appreciation of nature, music, art, and many other things. And, as has been discussed in this book, older adults sustain many losses. The most vulnerable older adults—in terms of inability to adjust to losses—are those for whom life's meaning is centered in one activity or relationship. It is lovely to see a couple who is very deeply in love. But if this pair has made the other the sole source of soul in their lives, each is susceptible to despair after the other dies. It is so important for each individual to develop meaning in a number of ways so that the basket has a number of eggs, that the loss of one does not empty it.

For some, this may make one hesitant to love much. What's the point? If I love someone deeply, or apply myself fully to a calling or activity, and lose it, then I'm lost; I'm done; I'm finished! Some people never attach deeply to anything because of this reasoning, consciously or unconsciously.

But meaning is found in engagement. Social entrepreneur Jacqueline Novogratz (2010) said, "Our job in life is not to be perfect, but only to be human." She went on to develop her thesis that it is better to immerse oneself in the aspects of life that one chooses to expend oneself in than to live life "untouched." There is profound risk in loving, in engaging, in trying. But in the messiness of learning, of trying, of failing, and of succeeding (some people fear success as much as failure) is meaning.

And, of course, choosing to deeply involve oneself in certain areas means one has no time or energy for engagement with other things; there is a cost. This contrasts with the North American notion that if you dream big, you can have it or do it. Popular culture is not always accurate, and this uniquely western idea is simply not true. To truly immerse ourselves—to choose one of life's options—means that we "unchoose" another. Mature adults accept that responsibility and make peace with it.

As an older adult, choose to engage as deeply as your resources (time, finances, health, energy) allow you to, and make sure that your basket contains a number of eggs. It cannot contain more eggs than you can hold (to extend the metaphor), but carry, for as long as you can, a number of them.

LINE UP YOUR LIFE CHOICES WITH YOUR VALUES

At the beginning of this book, we described the concept of miswanting (Gilbert & Wilson, 2000). Miswanting, the mistaken belief that new objects, such as cars or jewelry, will bring happiness, can be more of a trap than we realize. We might believe that we foster our sense of meaning through involvement in church and doing good deeds for others, but spend significant time shopping, wanting, and buying objects and talking about and showing these objects. Although we believe we have attended to meaning in our lives, we feel empty. We may not recognize the misalignment of our beliefs in and focus on day-to-day living; when we redirect our wants to involve others less fortunate, we may unexpectedly discover what we were missing.

Considering how you spend your time is not a one-time event. From time to time, especially when you're feeling dissatisfied with life, it may be worthwhile to recheck how you spend your time. Have you drifted into too much television watching? Do your days lack structure and are you bored? Are you spending an inordinate amount of time in bed, not because of fatigue but because you cannot stand not knowing how to fill your day when awake?

PUT INTO PRACTICE SPIRITUAL PRACTICES

If we understand the word *spiritual* to broadly refer to the expression of a soul's passion, then the number of spiritual practices is countless. In the practice of the Christian faith, we hear about many disciplines: prayer, Scripture reading and memory, and church attendance. As so much has been written on these subjects, we will not specifically focus upon these. In this next section, we will focus on some spiritual disciplines that may not be as common, and that can make a wonderful difference in the final stages of your life's work of art.

WRESTING AND RESTING

As stated earlier, meaning-making involves wresting and resting. That is, part of making meaning is laborious and demands commitment and hard work. Wresting can mean serious thinking or doing. For instance, you might think seriously about what you can do to squeeze out meaning in your days, or you might set aside time every day to pray about it, asking God for direction. Additionally, it might involve doing, such as attending church, helping out a neighbor, or contributing to a cause that is in line with your beliefs and passions.

There are also times when meaning involves resting, times when we need to rest from our striving. The well-known Serenity Prayer by Reinhold Niebuhr reads:

God grant me the serenity
To accept the things I cannot change;
Courage to change the things I can;
And wisdom to know the difference.
(lords-prayer-words.com, 2016, italics ours)

Applying the Serenity Prayer, resting involves acceptance of what we cannot change. To rest is no small feat! For some, resting is far more difficult than wresting. The activity of wresting may help us in that we feel we are *doing something*. Resting feels like we are standing still— not doing a blessed thing. We suggest that sometimes resting takes more effort than wresting. When we put our beliefs and faith in action by resting in the providence of the Almighty, this is an active choice and one which we may often have to revisit.

As noted earlier, it can be difficult to know when to wrest and when to rest. In terms of the Serenity Prayer, this involves wisdom. How much wresting versus resting takes place in meaning-making is probably dependent upon the person, his or her circumstances, and individual personality. However, both are important in meaning-making. How so? An example from the world of running may be helpful.

Individuals who run marathons train hard and strategically. Runners who are truly committed to this sport frequently want to train seven days per week. Often, they are counseled to take a couple of days off from training each week. Some runners will feel like this is two days wasted when they could be enhancing their speed and endurance. They are advised to take these days off to allow their bodies to heal and repair. They may be taught to view these days as training, but training of a different sort. The rest is seen as integral to the success of working out (Stanton, 1999).

Similarly, resting from wresting is good for mental and spiritual health; we cannot always be striving towards goals. What does resting entail? Certainly, resting involves the physical and spiritual self. Physically, it may involve taking care of one's body: getting enough sleep and ensuring proper nutrition. Spiritually, resting can include prayer and reading Scripture and meditations congruent with our beliefs. Resting can also involve visiting with individuals who feed our souls through laughter, meaningful connection, shared history, and mutual interests.

Learning how to rest between periods of wresting is not easy. We confess that we are not good at resting! Periods between jobs have been difficult. Our souls are often restless and strive towards squeezing out meaning in our daily lives (wresting). In taking our own counsel, perhaps we need to consider times of resting as important as wresting, and recognize more the significance of praying and reflecting upon where we have been, are currently at, and where we are going.

Sometimes the loss is such that it is necessary to move, over time, from wresting to resting. For the older adult, the death of a spouse is one example. The wresting that occurs in the grieving process (such as Kubler-Ross's denial, bargaining, and anger) must eventually move to resting (akin to Kubler-Ross's acceptance). How does this happen? A short answer would be facile. However, from experience with people who have wrested and rested through great struggles, an *internal* shift often happens; this shift cannot be demanded by well-meaning others. ("Snap out of it; she's with the Lord!" generally is not helpful.) The striving gives way to quiescence; wresting becomes resting. *"Be still, and know that I am God"* (Psalm 46:10, KJV) becomes *"My grace is sufficient"* (2 Corinthians 12:9, KJV). The ability to do this is both a choice of the one who brings herself before God—an inner posture of rest, giving oneself to the Lord—and the grace given by God to trust. Both a discipline and a gift, learning to rest when one has wrested is spiritual muscle to cope with the losses of older age.

Monitor Self-Talk

Earlier, we highlighted the study of Dwyer and colleagues (2008) in regards to finding meaning in a nursing home. The importance of self-talk was stressed. What we say to ourselves—about ourselves—is critical for meaning and purpose. The monitoring of self-talk can be considered a spiritual discipline because right thinking builds us up spiritually, and the monitoring of this internal monologue is counseled in Scripture. The Apostle Paul spoke to the Corinthians about this discipline: *"fitting every loose thought and emotion and impulse into the structure of life shaped by Christ"* (2 Corinthians 10:5, The Message). This can be hard work! It involves catching thoughts that are despairing, destructive, and false from a scriptural perspective, and refocusing on that which is true. A very famous passage illustrates this well:

> *Summing it all up, friends, I'd say you'll do best by filling your minds and meditating on things true, noble, reputable, authentic, compelling, gracious—the best, not the worst; the beautiful, not the ugly; things to praise, not things to curse. Put into practice what you learned from me, what you heard and saw and realized. Do that, and God, who makes everything work together, will work you into his most excellent harmonies.*
> —Philippians 4:8–9, The Message

When we reinforce ideas that we are no longer of any use in this world through unhealthy self-talk, meaning in life will be lost and despair will ensue. However, when we can remember who we are as individuals and reinforce within our inner dialogue aspects of a character we prize, we may begin to see ways in which we still express these characteristics, even in drastically different circumstances.

For instance, the older adult who ran marathons for decades but now cannot run, and even finds walking painful, may not be able to express his dogged determination through running long distances, but he may still express that rugged fortitude through living independently, applying himself at work (volunteer or paid), and even working his upper body at the gym. Thus his circumstances have markedly changed, but his indomitable spirit remains and may even be expressed to a greater degree than when he was fully able. This can bring great meaning; his strong independence and fortitude have been fueled by inner dialogue that stresses capability.

For the man who is caring for a wife suffering from dementia, monitoring self-talk is absolutely essential. His efforts are enormous, the energy expended huge; it would be very easy for him to descend into an inner dialogue that is critical—of his spouse and of himself. Those around him do not see the amount of work involved in this care; he is reticent to speak to others about it, as he wants to guard her dignity. There is no cheering section. Oh, but wait, perhaps there is!

O Lord, you have examined my heart
and know everything about me.
You know when I sit down or stand up.
You know my thoughts even when I'm far away.
You see me when I travel
and when I rest at home.
You know everything I do.
You know what I am going to say
even before I say it, Lord.
You go before me and follow me.
You place your hand of blessing on my head.
Such knowledge is too wonderful for me,
too great for me to understand!
I can never escape from your Spirit!
I can never get away from your presence!
                                        —Psalm 139:1–7, NLT

This gentleman is not alone in his struggle; there is One who sees and knows, and this divine knowledge is wonderful (139:6) because it assures him of his Lord's care. As God knows each thought, this may be the impetus for him to monitor his self-talk; it *does* matter, not just to his wife and himself, but to the loving One who is ever before him and following, too (Psalm 139:5). And his life, while lived largely in secret, is not useless; it is priceless to the King who says, *"Truly, I say to you, as you did it to the [most vulnerable], you did it me"* (Matthew 25:40, RSV). When the time comes that this man needs to place his wife in a nursing home, he will continue to care for her, and the One who watches over this couple will continue to care for both of them.

SELF-TRANSCENDENCE

In Chapter Two, we addressed the concept of self-transcendence. We discussed how this concept involves the expansion of one's boundaries to include an inward focus, an outward focus, and the element of time. In this discussion, we gave examples of what the expression of self-transcendence involves (according to Reed, 2009).

The benefit of understanding the multi-dimensional concept of self-transcendence lies not just in the variety of activities that can address introspection, outward focus, and perspectives across time, but also in that we can adapt our pursuit of meaning according to our life circumstances. If we are convalescing from surgery at home, we may not be able to volunteer at an animal shelter for that time; however, we can enjoy nature outside, read a book that speaks to our souls, call a friend who is lonely, or pray. All of these actions address the introspective aspect of self-transcendence, or the outward focus, but in a different fashion.

Marlette was privileged to see a spontaneous example of self-transcendence—particularly drawing from the past to make meaning in the present (Reed, 2009)—some years ago. While visiting a very elderly lady in a nursing home, she heard a musical group perform in the common room. The elderly woman, Rhonda, had been an actress and dancer for many years. In her older years, she was not able to participate in the profession; physical disabilities and cognitive issues made this impossible. As Rhonda and Marlette came into the common room, the seats at the back were all taken and she had to move to the very front to get a seat. So, with her walker ahead of her, she journeyed to the front of the room. The band saw her coming and began to encourage her with an upbeat number and clapping. Right at the front, Rhonda transcended her circumstances and was transported to another time: with a wiggle and the raising of arms, she did a little dance for the band and the crowd. The audience erupted with applause, and Rhonda was again the dancer on the stage. A beautiful example! The ability to adapt our meaning-making activities to our life, health, and environmental circumstances will provide stability in changes that occur with aging.

From a spiritual perspective, self-transcendence could be compared to Jesus' instruction to lose our lives so that we may gain them (see Luke 9:24–26). Giving up our right to control is not a sign of weakness as it is sometimes understood; the person who has no sense of self and so never makes decisions and never seizes the day is not one who has "lost their life" for Jesus' sake, or the sake of others. Rather, true self-transcendence, losing so that one may gain, is the choice of the person who knows themselves, exercises healthy control in their lives (remember, self-control is a fruit of the Spirit), and releases that control in trust of God when circumstances warrant it. Releasing control and turning one's spirit to other thoughts and endeavors frees one who cannot do what once was their practice.[8] In a different expression of the spirit, soul, and self, that person is able to experience meaning that is truly otherworldly. Using our earlier example of the gentleman caring for his wife with dementia, his losing his life for her is truly self-transcendent.

FORGIVENESS

No one gets through life without hurting others or being hurt by others, and the concept of forgiveness is touched upon in various places in this book. Hence, a chapter about putting it all together would not be complete without inserting this vital spiritual discipline. What is forgiveness? It is the choice of the wounded individual to release the hurt and the wounding individual in order to move on. While we tend to think that forgiveness means that the wounding person gets off free, the internal act of forgiveness actually releases the forgiving individual. Carrying the hurt(s) another has inflicted upon our souls is a great weight, and it takes a tremendous amount of energy, with no positive outcome. Perspective is lost, as one's focus remains glued to the offense(s); the offending individual may not even recognize that they have caused this harm. Lewis Smedes, who wrote extensively on the

---

8 One could say that self-transcendence at its greatest expression occurs when people give up what we would consider human rights—like freedom—and transcend, rise above those circumstances through differing activities and through relationship with the Transcendent.

topic of forgiveness, said, "To forgive is to set a prisoner free and discover that the prisoner was you" (Brainy Quotes, 2016f).

What does forgiveness involve? Smedes (2001) spoke of several components to this discipline. First, one gives up his right to get even with the offending individual; the eye-for-an-eye principle is released. Second, the one who has been hurt rediscovers the humanity in the one who has hurt them. It is so easy to demonize the wounding individual, not simply because we have been hurt, but also because actions against us can be evil! And third, Smedes said that forgiveness involves wishing the offender well. As Jesus counseled, we are to bless those who curse us (Luke 6:27–29).

This sounds like a tall order—and for the major offenses in our lives, it is. In the context of being a spiritual discipline, the muscles of forgiveness truly get built up as we live lives of releasing people—and hence ourselves—from others' offenses.

For Marlette, as a chaplain at the bedside of countless dying individuals, the issue of forgiveness has often come up. One man said about forgiveness within his fractured family, "Sometimes it's just too late." If one has worked the spiritual muscles throughout one's life, he is more likely to be able to forgive towards the end. This counsel is not meant to whack on the head those who take the concern of forgiveness seriously. There are those who may struggle to forgive all their lives, and the struggle alone works the spiritual muscle. Smedes (2001) mentioned that English scholar and theologian C.S. Lewis struggled his entire life to forgive a harsh school master; at the end of his life, Lewis felt that he had, perhaps, finally done it. Smedes wryly noted that if Lewis had lived longer, he would have probably needed to forgive this man again! The merit is in the spiritual discipline that involves the actions and attitudes described by Smedes (2001) above. The direction of the heart is the most important thing.

And has been noted earlier, to forgive does not mean one must get back into relationship. Relationship involves trust, and it may not be wise to trust the one who has deeply wounded you; a healthy relationship is predicated upon safety. God sees and knows the heart which does the spiritual work of forgiving.

To forgive others allows us to free ourselves, free up our thoughts to think upon other things, and conserve our emotions for those activities which have a positive payoff. From the perspective of the self, it aids the self. It is also self-transcending, as described earlier; those who have been truly able to self-transcend in history are those who have been able to forgive, such as Corrie and Betsie ten Boom, in a women's concentration camp in World War 2. It is also what Jesus did at Calvary: *"'Father, forgive these peo- ple,' Jesus said, 'for they don't know what they are doing.... Father, I commit my spirit to you'"* (Luke 23:34, 46, TLB).

SPIRITUAL REMINISCENCE

Reminiscence and spiritual reminiscence are forms of therapy for older adults in which they are invited to think about their lives and recall and relate memories of them- selves. Often, this occurs with a nurse or recreational ther- apist in a group setting, such as a mental health unit or nursing home unit. With reminiscence therapy, the group leader may introduce an artifact, such as a weaving loom, and invite members to speak about what they know about the loom, whether they ever used this apparatus or have memories about one. The use of reminiscence can be very powerful to pull the older adult out of the present—which may be marred by memory loss or mental illness—into the past, which may feel safer.

Annette has witnessed the powerful effect this type of therapy can have on older adults. In one instance, an older gentleman, who was quite paranoid and for the most part refused to speak, became very animated, lively, and talkative as he described an object from the past. The object allowed him to tap into memories that were a safe and secure place for him.

Spiritual reminiscence is similar to reminiscence, but there is a greater emphasis upon meaning. As such, spiritual reminiscence is a way in which older adults can reflect upon their lives and tell stories about their past, but do so with an emphasis of meaning (MacKinlay & Trevitt, 2010). The group facilitator will ask questions of members, thus inviting individuals to think more deeply about their lives. By retelling their life stories, issues of grief, anger, loss, and joy can be accessed. Past experiences can be reframed so that they are viewed in a new light, thereby bringing peace and a sense of resolution (MacKinlay & Trevitt, 2010).

> Spiritual reminiscence is a way in which older adults can reflect upon their lives and tell stories about their past, but do so with an emphasis of meaning.

We believe that spiritual reminiscence can be conducted formally within a group with a trained facilitator, or informally in a self-review. If you are reflecting upon your life within the privacy of your home, considering what has brought meaning and joy as well as spiritual and emotional pain, and find it difficult to move beyond this, then consulting a professional, such as a chaplain or minister, or a mental health professional would be helpful. Sometimes we reflect upon regrets, sadness, and perceived failures and are unable to grant to ourselves the same grace that we might extend to others. Having an outside person listen to our stories and offer alternate ways of understanding our past circumstances and actions can truly be freeing!

If you are reflecting upon your life and what has brought meaning, it can remind you of times in your life that were particularly good. This allows you to consider, "What was good about that time? What was I doing that was so meaningful or good?" This may give you clues about what you were thinking, feeling, or doing differently in the past that worked for you, and which you have now unwittingly let slip. This may prompt you to consider how you can change your thinking and actions, and thus enhance meaning in your life.

This kind of reminiscence is vital in putting together the pieces of one's life. If there are things to be corrected, steps can be taken to correct them. The individual who is reminiscing can be assisted by a professional to identify themes of their lives and recognize the contribution they have made. This is vital spiritual work! Where there are loose and frayed threads in the tapestry, efforts can be made to address them, weaving these frayed threads back into the masterpiece. And the beauty of the tapestry can be affirmed by someone who stands apart from the individual.

Annette M. Lane and Marlette B. Reed

GRAB HOLD OF THE REDEMPTIVE
THREADS OF YOUR TAPESTRY

A theme related to but not the same as spiritual reminiscence is God reclaiming the ills suffered in this life to bring forth good things. There is a lovely redemptive thread that weaves itself throughout the pages of the Scriptures. From the get-go, there was trouble in fallen creation. Evil happened to people who did not deserve it, tragedies occurred, sometimes the tragedies transpired from one's own making, and other times they arose from the avarice of others. But from the book of Genesis forward, there is a theme that is emphasized throughout: God can bring forth beauty out of ugliness. This does not mean that the ugliness is good, but that beauty, in itself impossible without the ugliness, may be brought forth.

In the Old Testament, this truth is enunciated particularly clearly in the words of Joseph, who after confronting his brothers on their selling him into slavery (and all that happened as a result of that catalyst) said, *"Now don't be worried or angry with yourselves because you sold me here. God sent me here ahead of you to save people's lives"* (Genesis 45:5, NCV, emphasis ours). Later, the Apostle Paul says, *"Moreover we know that to those who love God, who are called according to his plan, everything that happens fits into a pattern for good"* (Romans 8:28, Phillips).

It is too easy to allow the evils we have experienced to define us permanently as damaged. And unfortunately, we live in that mistaken belief as prisoners of the if-onlys. ("If only that had never happened, I'd be in a different place, I'd be a different person.") The Scriptures let us know that God uses everything in this broken world to form us into the beautiful image of His Son (Romans 8:29), who also had evil inflicted upon Him. And through this, He redeemed and reclaimed us!

Can you look at the events in your life that you wish had never happened and see some thread of redemption in it? We in no way mean to minimize what you have experienced, but one's understanding of suffering strongly impacts a sense of meaning in one's life. Writer Andrew Solomon (2014) spoke movingly about a woman who had been raped in her teens, which resulted in a pregnancy and a child. This now fifty-year-old woman indicated that she used to think of her assailant with anger, but now just with pity. Why? Because, she said, this man does not know that he has a wonderful daughter and grandchildren—and she does. From that event, she has done what Andrew Solomon termed "forging meaning." And she has done so, much in the same way that Joseph and the Apostle Paul designated meaning to the events of their lives. To alter the metaphor, the jagged pieces of her life have been brought together into a vase with seams of gold and silver that reflect beautifully her love, grace, and courage.

> It is never too late to grab hold of the redemptive thread of God's creative hand in our lives.

It is never too late to grab hold of the redemptive thread of God's creative hand in our lives. Your suffering, perhaps even the suffering you inflicted and then regretted, has worked together in the Weaver's fingers to knit together a unique work of art. Recognizing this will bring peace; it will also allow you to cooperate with the Lord in the work of your life, redefining yourself as you are seen by your Maker—one who bears the image of Christ.

SEEK OUT FELLOW SOJOURNERS IN THE PURSUIT OF MEANING

It is meaningful to discuss our pursuit of meaning with other like-minded people! This can occur while walking, over a cup of coffee, or while relaxing in a backyard on a warm summer's day. Others can add insights we have not considered and challenge us to think more deeply or perhaps less deeply (for those prone to morbid introspection). A dialogue can focus on concepts, but in the area of meaning, these concepts will naturally become personal, and the two individuals can help each other in understanding weaknesses as well as strengths, areas of fear as well as faith, supporting each other in this walk. As Proverbs 27:17 says, *"iron sharpens iron"* (NIV).

RELATIONSHIP WITH GOD

This brief section will not attempt to cover such a broad topic in few words; rather, relationship with God will be approached from an end-of-life perspective, completing the masterpiece.

ETERNITY IN OUR HEARTS

The first quote in this book was the statement from the book of Ecclesiastes that God has set eternity in our hearts (3:11). As folks get older and the pace of life slows, so often their hearts turn towards ultimate meanings. "Am I ready to meet my Maker? Will I see loved ones who have passed away again? What does heaven look like?"

There are a plethora of books about near-death experiences and encounters on "the other side," and so there is no need to go into these subjects in depth here. Suffice it to say, there is something in the human heart that believes in an afterlife; while at the grave we may say "ashes to ashes, dust to dust," the essence of a person, her spirit, lives on. The Eternal One who breathed life into humanity has set that conviction in the human heart.

And so it is natural that as people age (or, in the case of terminal illness, those who are not aged but rather very sick), their thoughts turn towards God. How beautiful it is to witness this! Every Christian denomination has its forms for conversion, recommitment, and preparation for death, but the form is not nearly as important as the heart's turning. From her work with dying people, Marlette has become convinced that God is very involved in preparing people for their final transition.

As one's heart turns towards God, the issue of the need for forgiveness may come up. In such cases, the individual knows within themselves what they need to bring to God. Many denominations have forms for confession, which can be helpful. But as in our discussion on forgiving others, the form is not nearly as important as the intent of the heart. If a simple form is desired, the Lord's Prayer (Luke 11:2–4) contains all the theology a person could need in terms of recognizing the supremacy of God, asking for help and forgiveness of sins and giving God glory.

Annette M. Lane and Marlette B. Reed

Fears About Getting Safely to the Other Side

So many sincere, devout people fear getting from A to B in the ultimate sense—transitioning from life on earth to heaven. And so, a few fears and responses to those fears will be touched upon here.

First, people fear that God may not be good, and may not love them. Dying is the ultimate release of control, transcending from one realm to another. Fears from childhood teaching are often behind this: "If you do bad things, you will spend eternity in hell." The remedy to this, of course, is the understanding that we belong to God, the price for sin has been paid, and God loves us completely.

However, for sensitive souls who received teaching that emphasized judgment, the programming on the hard drive can be difficult to edit. Marlette worked with a dear Christian lady, Jenny, who feared that when she crossed over, she would not receive Jesus' *"Well done, thou good and faithful servant"* (Matthew 25:21, KJV). Jenny did not have any outstanding things to make right, she was walking closely with the Lord, but she was venturing into unknown territory (dying), which activated the programming on her hard drive (that fear that, no matter what, she would not be good enough for God). Marlette worked with her from the Scriptures, and from a perspective of monitoring her thoughts. When they spoke about these things, Jenny was helped; however, when she was alone at night, she struggled. Marlette encouraged her to have scriptures ready for those times when she was alone and anxious.

Some people think that if they have fear, they obviously don't believe. (Have we not all been told that fear is the opposite of faith?) These folks become disappointed in themselves that they are more anxious as they age, particularly as they approach their latter years and perhaps days. However, it is very natural to have more anxiety as we age. For example, fear often comes with cognitive impairment, whether that impairment is due to dementia or brain cancer. As well, it is natural to fear the unknown, and crossing over is the ultimate unknown. Folks have often asked Marlette, "What is it like on the other side?" And she has had to say, "I'm sorry, I've never been!" So if you are finding yourself anxious, be gracious with yourself. If you have some physical issues, these may be exacerbating your fear. Don't be afraid to speak with your doctor about your concerns.

Some sensitive souls fear that in "crossing the Jordan" (whose waters are chilly and cold), they may drown. Or, to switch the metaphor, when the chariot swings low, "coming for to carry me home," said chariot may swing low but miss them entirely! To this fear, there is an incredibly comforting scripture: *"Precious in the sight of the Lord is the death of his saints"* (Psalm 116:15, KJV). Not only is the physical passing precious, but the dying process also. If the dying process is so precious, will not our Lord carefully swing that chariot low and accurately?

(RE)TURNING TO GOD AT END OF LIFE: IS THIS DISINGENUOUS?

This question is sometimes asked by people who have been raised with faith but did not practice it during their adult years. It is also asked by those who have not ever practiced faith and are worried about what others may think, even what God may think, as they call out to Him in the foxhole.

The Scriptures make it very clear that the main issue is not when the turn/return happens, but that it does happen. The prodigal son received an over-the-top welcome from his father, even after having squandered his father's wealth (see Luke 15:11–32). Other titles that have been suggested for this parable are *The Lost Son, The Running Father,* and *The Lovesick Father.* How meaningful are these other titles for the parable of Prodigal Son! The son has been lost (he is not wicked); the father is not staid (he thrusts aside his dignity and runs toward his son). The father is not emotionally cool; with his son's absence, he has been lovesick! Such is the case with the elderly one who begins to approach her Heavenly Father. She is received with open arms, welcomed, celebrated!

Going back to the idea of foxhole religion, C.S. Lewis (in Moore, 2015) spoke about what war does in people's lives. He stated the following in an address to students at Oxford just weeks after the outbreak of World War II:

> *What does war do to death? It certainly does not make it more frequent; 100 percent of us die, and the percentage cannot be increased... Yet war does do something to death. It forces us to remember it. War makes death real to us...*

It is the reality of death that turns one's thoughts towards God; and in a foxhole, one naturally thinks about death. As the aged recognize that their energies are limited, and so more carefully determine their activities, they understand that death and the afterlife are coming. It is from this perspective that they begin to turn inward.

In conjunction with life processes and stages, Marlette believes that the Holy Spirit "works overtime" on those who are approaching life's end. The Counselor, the Comforter, the Revealer of Truth, the One who groans within us, the Good Spirit prepares us for the final transition. Going back to Psalm 116:15, precious in the sight of the Lord—in the sight of the Lovesick Father, Emmanuel ("God with us"), and the Comforter—is the passing of one set apart (a saint).

Jenny, in her dying process, was somnolent for days. She experienced what we would term today as deathbed phenomena—or, to put it another way, she had one foot in heaven and one foot still on earth. In her somnolence, she would occasionally open her eyes and exclaim "Glorious!" Marlette believes that Jenny, who feared not getting the "well done" from her Savior, was treated to glimpses of heaven and of Jesus in her dying, to help her cross over gently. She said "Glorious!" in her glimpses. And the staff of the palliative care ward who watched this happen over the course of several days whispered "Glorious!" and "Holy" as they witnessed her passing.

PUTTING IT ALL TOGETHER

How does one's life become a masterpiece in older age? Likely, your life is already a masterpiece in certain ways, and has room for touch ups in other ways (the human condition).

First, take stock by looking at the past. Having one who can help you with this—a friend or a pastor or counselor—may aid you, particularly if you need help reframing things, as the very sensitive often do, or if there is something particularly traumatic you wish to look at. Don't be afraid to write things down in a journal, perhaps titled *My Life: A Work of Art*—it's your choice whether it's a tapestry, a vase, or a painting! Writing these things down will help you to make them concrete, less wispy. On days when you question the value of your earthly contribution, go back to this journal; let the notations encourage you!

For the areas that are not at masterpiece level, do what you can to rectify things. This may mean saying "I'm sorry," reconnecting with a good friendship that died from neglect, or fulfilling dreams that are still possible. This does not mean obsessively turning over every stone of your life, in case you may have hurt someone. Rather, for the things that come up naturally in your heart and mind in quiet moments, seek to address them. By doing this, you may grab hold of meaning that both blesses you and others. You may wish to write down these regrets and what you did to rectify them.

And finally, practice the spiritual disciplines spoken of in this book, and others that you already possess. These disciplines will powerfully impact your internal life. Remember A.J. Jacobs? In his year of "living biblically," he took from that experience the need to be a grateful person.

> *Another lesson is that thou shalt give thanks... I was praying, giving these prayers of thanksgiving, which was odd for an agnostic. But I was saying thanks all the time, every day, and I started to change my perspective.... So, this is actually a key to happiness for me...* (Jacobs, 2008)

In your work-of-art journal, you may also record some results of your spiritual disciplines, such as keeping record of things to be grateful for and answers to prayer. Each journal will be as unique as the person writing in it.

One last point about such a history: your history can be passed along to your children and grandchildren, if you choose, as a glimpse into your life. It can be a priceless gift! When the grandmother of Marlette's husband passed, he received an invaluable present: her Bible. This deeply devout woman stored in her Bible her history of faith, prayer, and life in the pages of this deeply worn book. Prayer requests from others, her notations penciled in the margins, service bulletins from weddings and funerals, spiritual steps written down—these filled the pages. Marlette and Brian spent much time going through this copy of the Scriptures, as it gave them insight into a woman they treasured.

On a similar note, Marlette officiated at the funeral for a woman who had suffered deep trauma in her childhood. This particular trauma, which she believed she had caused (an accident), she carried deeply within herself all her life. In the months before her death, she compiled a written history of her life, in which she addressed this. Oh, the gift that this chronicle of her life was to her adult children! They understood her on a whole different level; they appreciated her ability to continue in her life and to raise her seven children (a feat all its own, but particularly noteworthy with the heavy emotional load she bore all her life), and they cherished this end-of-life recollection as a means by which she could be remembered by them and their children.

Whether or not you choose such a tangible expression of the masterpiece of your life, or whether you wish to get from A to B without permanent record, know that your work will impact you and those who love you meaningfully.

QUESTIONS TO PONDER:

- How does my faith help me in my pursuit for meaning?
- As I age, what facets of meaning can I develop further? What aspects do I need assistance with from family or my church family?
- Are there events in my life that need revisiting, to forge different meaning from them? How does this new meaning impact how I view myself and my life?

TIPS FOR CONSIDERATION:

- Begin a journal in which you document meaningful aspects of each day. This may help you to look for meaning in the everyday, including the mundane or unexpected.
- Journal about where you would like to go in your pursuit of meaning and what needs to happen to bring this to fruition.
- If you have done work from other chapters, add this work into this journal in a creative way.

Afterword

Is not wisdom found among the aged? Does not long life bring understanding? To God belong wisdom and power; counsel and understanding are his.

—Job 12:12–13 (NIV)

Youth is happy because it has the capacity to see beauty. Anyone who keeps the ability to see beauty never grows old.

—Franz Kafka
Author
(Quotations Page, 2016)

Thank you for sojourning through this territory of meaning with us! While we have written the book over a number of months, discussing concepts as we walked, passing the manuscript back and forth as we developed and redeveloped ideas, really, this book is the culmination of years of wresting and resting with meaning in our lives. In our teenage years and early adulthood, we often felt alone as we wrestled with existential issues even within our faith paradigm, as our friends and counterparts seemed oblivious to such angst. Interestingly, as we have entered our fifties, we find ourselves less lonely; more of our generation is experiencing similar issues and seeking meaning in their lives. And as we have experienced health challenges, as well as the deaths of our parents and other family members, the concepts related to meaning-making, such as self-transcendence, have come alive for us.

As we finish this work, Annette had the beautiful experience of chatting with a very elderly gentleman in a parking lot. Annette is prone to chatting with people everywhere, particularly if they have dogs! This gentleman was very sad as he showed her his massive dog that would be euthanized later that day (the animal was very sick). This gentleman was taking out Jupiter for his last meal—a burger. As this fellow talked with Annette, he sobbed. The conversation lasted for just ten minutes, but he was consoled. At the end, there was a hug and many thanks from this elderly man.

The meaning in this incident came about through their shared humanity; both had lost dogs, both care for animals and for those who love them, and both know the loneliness that comes from losing a cherished companion. There was a sense of the Sacred and this gentleman would have gone home with his burden lightened just a little bit. Both experienced a sense that they were in this life together. Marlette feels strongly that Emmanuel, who knew life's losses and loneliness too, was pleased. The connection between Annette and this grieving gentleman in a parking lot infused her day with life's essence; meaning is to be found everywhere, if only one has their spiritual lenses focused.

We wish you all the best as you consider meaning in your life and what it means to you to have meaning, pursue meaning, and sustain meaning throughout your aging years.

References

Bradley Bursack, C. (2015). "Do parents really want to live with their adult children?" *AgingCare.com*. Retrieved on May 9, 2016 from https://www.agingcare.com/Articles/parents-living-with-adult-children-152285.htm

Brainy Quotes. (2016a). Viktor E. Frankl quotes. Retrieved April 24, 2016 from http://www.brainyquote.com/quotes/authors/v/viktor_e_frankl.html

Brainy Quotes. (2016b). C.S. Lewis quotes. Retrieved April 24, 2016 from http://www.brainyquote.com/quotes/authors/c/c_s_lewis_3.html

Brainy Quotes. (2016c). Sue Monk Kidd quotes. Retrieved May 16, 2016 from http://www.brainyquote.com/quotes/authors/s/sue_monk_kidd.html

Brainy Quotes. (2016d). Mundane quotes. Retrieved April 21, 2016 from http://www.brainyquote.com/quotes/keywords/mundane.html

Brainy Quotes. (2016e). Socrates quotes. Retrieved May 13, 2016 from http://www.brainyquote.com/quotes/quotes/s/socrates101168.html

Brainy Quotes (2016f). Lewis B. Smedes quotes. Retrieved June 27, 2016 from http://www.brainyquote.

com/quotes/quotes/l/lewisbsme135524.html?s-rc=t_forgive

Bute, J. (2016). My glorious opportunity: How my dementia has been a gift. *Journal of Religion, Spirituality, & Aging, 28*(1/2), 15–23.

Damianakis, T., & Marziali, E. (2012). Older adults' response to the loss of a spouse: The function of spirituality in understanding the grieving process. *Aging & Mental Health, 16* (1), 57–66.

Drury, M. (1988). The last half of life. *Reader's Digest,* November, 105–107.

Dwyer, L-L., Nordenfelt, L., & Ternestedt, B-M. (2008). Three nursing home residents speak about meaning at the end of life. *Nursing Ethics, 15*(1), 97–109. doi: 10.1177/0969733007083938

Efron, N. (2008). *I feel bad about my neck: And other thoughts about being a woman.* New York, NY: Vintage.

Ersner-Hershfield, H., Mikels, J.A., Sullivan, S.J., & Carstensen, L.L. (2008). Poignancy: Mixed emotional experience in the face of meaningful endings. *Journal of Personality and Social Psychology, 94*(1), 158–167.

Evidence Network. (2012). Why seniors matter—and how they contribute to our everyday lives. Retrieved May 04, 2016 from http://umanitoba.ca/outreach/evidencenetwork/archives/7321

Franz Kafka Online. (2016). Franz Kafka quotes. Retrieved April 24, 2016 from http://www.kafka-online.info/franz-kafka-quotes.htm

Fredrickson, B.L., & Carstensen, L.L (1998). Choosing social partners: How old age and anticipated endings make people more selective. In L.M. Powell and T. Salthouse (Eds.), *Essential papers on the psychology of aging* (pp. 511–538). New York, NY: New York University Press.

Free Online Dictionary. (2016). Definition of mundane. Retrieved December 8, 2016 from http://www.thefreedictionary.com/mundane

Furnham, A. (2014). The dark side of happiness: Can happiness be bad for you? *Psychology Today,* Feb. 14. Retrieved May 8, 2016 from https://www.psychologytoday.com/blog/sideways-view/201402/the-dark-side-happiness

Gawande, A. (2014). *Being mortal: Medicine and what matters in the end.* New York, NY: Metropolitan Books.

Gilbert, D., & Wilson, T. (2000). Miswanting: Some problems in the forecasting of future affective states. In J.P. Forgas (Ed.), *Feeling and thinking: The role of affect in social cognition* (pp. 178-197). New York, NY: Cambridge University Press.

Glassner, B. (1999). *The culture of fear: Why Americans are afraid of the wrong things.* New York, NY: Basic Books.

Glassner, B. (2009). *The culture of fear: Why Americans are afraid of the wrong things—Updated for our post 9/11 world.* New York, NY: Basic Books.

Goodreads. (2016a). Morrie Schwartz—Quotes. Retrieved April 24, 2016 from https://www.goodreads.com/author/quotes/93035.Morrie_Schwartz

Goodreads. (2016b). Viktor E. Frankl—Quotes. Retrieved April 24, 2016 from http://www.goodreads.com/author/quotes/2782.Viktor_E_Frankl?page=4

Goodreads. (2016c). Quotes about meaning of life. Retrieved April 24, 2016 from http://www.goodreads.com/quotes/tag/meaning-of-life

Goodreads (2016d). Elisabeth Kubler-Ross quotes. Retrieved June 27, 2016 from http://www.goodreads. com/quotes/202404-the-most-beautiful-people-we-have-known-are-those-who

Goodreads. (2016e). Maya Angelou quotes. Retrieved April 29, 2016 from http://www.goodreads.com/ quotes/8639-i-ve-learned-that-regardless-of-your-relationship-with-your-parents

Groot-Alberts, L. (2012). The lament of a broken heart: mourning and grieving in different cultures. How acceptance of difference creates a bridge for healing and hope. *Progress in Palliative Care, 20*(3), 158–162.

Gunther, M. (2008). Deferred empathy: A construct with implications for the mental health of older adults. *Issues in Mental Health Nursing, 29*(9), 1029–1040. doi: 10.1080/01612840802274974

Haugan, G. (2014a). Meaning-in-life in nursing-home patients: A correlate to physical and emotional symptoms. *Journal of Clinical Nursing, 23*(7/8), 1030–1043.

Haugan, G. (2014b). Meaning-in-life in nursing-home patients: A valuable approach for enhancing psychological and physical well-being? *Journal of Clinical Nursing, 23*, 1830–1844. doi: 10.1111/jocn.12402

Haugan, G., Rannestad, T., Hammervold, R., Garasen, H., & Espnes, G. (2013). Self-transcendence in cognitively-impaired nursing-home patients: A resource for well being. *Journal of Advanced Nursing, 69*(5),1147–1160. doi: 10.1111/j.1365-2648.2012.06106.x

Honigman, R. & Castle, D.J. (2006). Aging and cosmetic enhancement. *Clinical Interventions in Aging, 1*(2), 115–119. Retrieved on May 9, 2015 from http://www. ncbi.nlm.nih.gov/pmc/articles/PMC2695163/

Jacobs, A.J. (2008). My year of living biblically. *TEDtalks.* Subtitles and Transcript retrieved on June 27, 2016 at https://www.ted.com/talks/a_j_jacobs_year_of_living_biblically/transcript?language=en

Jonsen, E., Norberg, A., & Lundman, B. (2015). Sense of meaning in life among the oldest old people living in a rural area of Sweden. *International Journal of Older People Nursing, 10*, 221-229. Doi: 10.1111/opn.12077

Kashdan, T. (2010). The problem with happiness. *Huffington Post.* Retrieved May 8, 2016 from http://www.huffingtonpost.com/todd-kashdan/whats-wrong-with-happines_b_740518.html

Lane, A.M., & Reed, M.B. (2015). *Older adults: Understanding and facilitating transitions* (2nd ed.). Dubuque, IA: Kendall Hunt.

lords-prayer-words.com. (2016). The serenity prayer. Retrieved May 02, 2016 from http://www.lords-prayer-words.com/famous_prayers/god_grant_me_the_serenity.html

MacKinlay, E., & Trevitt, C. (2016). Journeys with those who have dementia: Connecting and finding meaning in their journey. *Journal of Religion, Spirituality, & Aging, 28*(1/2), 24–36.

MacKinlay, E. (2010). Living in aged care: Using spiritual reminiscence to enhance meaning in life for those with dementia. *International Journal of Mental Health Nursing, 19*, 394–401.

Merriam-Webster. (2016). Definition of mentor. Retrieved December 8, 2016 from http://www.merriam-webster.com/dictionary/mentor

Moore, N. (2015). What do we make of finding religion in foxholes? *The Drum,* April 23. Retrieved on June 30,

2016 from http://www.abc.net.au/news/2015-04-24/ moore-what-do-we-make-of-finding-religion-in-foxholes/6415738

Morgan, J., & Farsides, T. (2009). Measuring meaning in life. *Journal of Happiness Studies, 10*, 197–214.

Novogratz, J. (2010). Inspiring a life of immersion. *TED-Women*. Annotated captions retrieved on June 22, 2016 from https://dotsub.com/view/22326cd2-cbc6-4b20-93e6-4e167b4ac12b/viewTranscript/eng

Pew Research Center. (2014). Multigenerational households. Retrieved December 8, 2016 from http://www. pewsocialtrends.org/2014/07/17/in-post-recession-era-young-adults-drive-continuing-rise-in-multi-generational-living/

Plett, H. (2016). What it really means to hold space for someone. *Uplift,* May 8. Retrieved on June 20, 2016 from http://upliftconnect.com/hold-space/

Plumadore, J., & Muehlherr, S. (2009). The golden rule across the world's religions. Scoutinglife.ca, November/December, 10–11 . Retrieved December 9, 2016 from http://www.scouts.ca/sites/default/files/sl-Golden-Rule-Across-Religion.pdf

Power Thesaurus (2016). Retrieved December 9, 2016 from www.powerthesaurus.org

Quotations Page. (2016). Quotations by author—Franz Kafka. Retrieved April 24, 2016 from http://www. quotationspage.com/quotes/Franz_Kafka

Quotegarden.com (2016a). Quotations: Retirement. Retrieved May 18, 2016 from http://www.quotegarden. com/retirement.html

Quotegarden.com. (2016b). Quotations about helping and making a difference. Retrieved April 24, 2016 from http://www.quotegarden.com/helping.html

Quote Sea. (2016). Quotes about follow through. Retrieved June 20, 2016 from http://www.quotesea.com/quotes/with/follow-through

Raje, A. (2012). *Global perspectives on multigenerational households and intergenerational relations: An ILC Global Alliance Report.* Retrieved May 9, 2016 from http://www.ilc-alliance.org/index.php/reports

Reed, P.G. (1991). Toward a nursing theory of self-transcendence: Deductive reformulation using developmental theories. *Advances in Nursing Sciences, 13*(4), 64–77.

Reed, P.G. (2009). Demystifying self-transcendence for mental health nursing practice and research. *Archives of Psychiatric Nursing, 23*(5), 397–400.

Smedes, L.B. (2001). Keys to forgiving. *Christianity Today,* December 3. Retrieved on June 27, 2016 from http://www.christianitytoday.com/ct/2001/december3/42.73.html

Solomon, A. (2014). How the worst moments of our lives make us who we are. *TEDTalks,* March. Retrieved July 1, 2016 from https://www.ted.com/talks/andrew_solomon_how_the_worst_moments_in_our_lives_make_us_who_we_are?language=en#t-251854

Stanton, J. (1999). *Running: Start to finish.* Edmonton, AB: Lone Pine.

Thinkexist.com. (2016). John Dewey quotes. Retrieved April 24, 2016 from http://thinkexist.com/quotes/john_dewey/3.html

Toohey, A.M., McCormack, G.R., Doyle-Baker, P.K., Adams, C.L., & Rock, M.J. (2013). Dog walking and sense of community in neighbourhoods: Implications for promoting physical activity in adults 50 years and older. *Health and Place, 22,* 75–81.

topix.com. (2016). The measure of a civilization is how it treats its weakest members. Retrieved May 16, 2016 from http://www.topix.com/forum/city/caruthersville-mo/T82RNKGEAJ1BP1QS6

United Nations Population Fund (2012). *Ageing in the twenty-first century; A celebration and a challenge.* New York, NY: United Nations Population Fund and HelpAge India.

Van Tongeren, D., Green, J., Davis, D., Hook, J., & Hulsey, T. (2016). Prosociality enhances meaning in life. *The Journal of Positive Psychology, 11*(3), 225–236. doi: 10.1080/17439760.2015.1048814

Weingarten, K. (2012). Sorrow: A therapist's reflection on the inevitable and unknowable. *Family Process, 51*(4), 440–454.

White, R. (2016). People feel more secure walking with a dog: Studies. *Calgary Herald,* February 27. Retrieved on May 9, 2016 from http://www.pressreader.com/canada/calgary-herald/20160227/283184377